Surviving the Death of Your Ex

MANAGING THE GRIEF NO ONE TALKS ABOUT

Edited by Robyn Hass, MSW, MPH
and Robbie Davis-Floyd, PhD

Praeclarus Press, LLC

www.PraeclarusPress.com

Praeclarus Press, LLC
2504 Sweetgum Lane
Amarillo, Texas 79124 USA
806-367-9950
www.PraeclarusPress.com

DISCLAIMER
The information contained in this publication is advisory only and is not
intended to replace sound clinical judgment or individualized patient
care. The author disclaims all warranties, whether expressed or implied,
including any warranty as the quality, accuracy, safety, or suitability of
this information for any particular purpose.

ISBN: 9781939807281

Cover Design: Ken Tackett
Copy Editing: Chris Tackett
Acquisition & Development: Kathleen Kendall-Tackett
Layout & Design: Cornelia Georgiana Murariu
Operations: Scott Sherwood

From Robyn

*This book is dedicated to my husband, Joseph.
Thank you for never letting go of my hand or my
heart, for walking through the fire with us, and for
being there to stand in the gap when my faith
was tested most. I love you more than
you will ever know.*

*To Jarod. You are one of the bravest
young men I've ever met. I know you are destined
for great things, and I love you more than you can
ever imagine! I'm so proud to be your mom.*

*And to Karen, for offering grace, forgiveness,
and love in the midst of heartache and tragedy.
You have made our family whole, and I will
always deeply treasure our friendship.*

From Robbie

*I dedicate this book to my adored son, Jason,
who has bravely survived the death of his beloved
father, and who now, to his great credit, is carrying
out and fulfilling the many rich and worthy legacies
his father left to all of us.*

CONTENTS

Introduction: **Why We Chose To Create This Book**   1
        Robyn Hass and Robbie Davis-Floyd

PART 1 - SURVIVING THE DEATH OF YOUR EX: ROBYN'S STORY   5

Chapter 1   Hearing the News   7

Chapter 2   Reality Sets In   23

Chapter 3   Time to Say Goodbye   41

Chapter 4   Life Goes On...Without You   51

Chapter 5   Let Hope Arise   61

Chapter 6   Finding Balance   73

PART 2 - SURVIVORS' STORIES   91

Chapter 7   On Being an Ex-Wife When Your
             Ex-Husband Dies: What Is Your Place?
             Where is Your Space? (*Robbie Davis-Floyd*)   93

Chapter 8   Presence of an Absence (*Kirsten Dehner*)   113

Chapter 9   The Brutal Murder of Mr. Hyde (*Annette Birchard*)   143

Chapter 10   It Seemed Crazy Because It Was (*Carol Wheeler*)   171

Chapter 11   Reflections of an Ex-Wife-Turned-Widow
              (*Laurie Wimmer*)   185

Chapter 12   Unexpected Consequences (*Melanie*)   193

Chapter 13   Chiaroscuro (*Alyeshka Harmon*)   201

Chapter 14   Love Lives On (*Rima Star*)   217

Conclusion   The End Is Just the Beginning
              (*Robyn Hass and Robbie Davis-Floyd*)   235

APPENDICES   241

    Appendix 1 The Art of Grieving Gracefully
                (*Robbie Davis-Floyd*)   243

    Appendix 2 Resources for Surviving the Death
                of Your Ex (*Robyn Hass*)   255

BIOGRAPHIES   258

WHY WE CHOSE TO CREATE THIS BOOK

Robyn Hass and Robbie Davis-Floyd

D ear Reader, we have created this book because we were stunned at the difficulties we both experienced when our ex-husbands died, and at the lack of any kind of accessible advice about how to deal with those difficulties. We had to cope with our own grief in the face of sometimes tenuous relationships with our exes' families, and with the massive grief our children felt when their fathers died, in the face of those same relationships. It fell to Robyn to tell her young son about his father's death, and to do her best to comfort him and ease him through the shock. Robbie's older son had to tell *her* that his dad had died, yet could offer her little support because his own grief was so great. We both had to do our best to figure out what were our appropriate roles, if any, in the notification of friends, the funeral arrangements, the complicated negotiations with families no longer our own, and so much more.

As a trained and degreed therapist, Robyn was familiar with loss and grief, but nothing prepared her for the plethora of mixed emotions that surfaced after his death—emotions that no one talked about. As she searched for professional literature on the subject, she realized that very little existed, and what was published was almost completely unavailable to the general public. So she began writing a journal, which turned into the chapters that now constitute Part 1 of this book, in an attempt to process her own emotions and to use her experience to help others.

Robbie's significant other at the time was Alan Huber, who was a friend of Robyn's, and so when he found himself having to comfort Robbie while she cried after her ex died, he decided to connect us, thinking that we might be able to help and support each other. Robyn had been planning to write her own book, and since Alan had told her that Robbie was a good editor, she sent her chapters to Robbie. While reading them with deep empathy and compassion, Robbie realized that she too wanted to write about her experience of the death of her ex, and that perhaps others would as well?

Robyn welcomed that suggestion, and so together, we put out a call through our various networks, which resulted in the other chapters in this book. We were delighted to receive each and every one, and edited them through tears (and sometimes, blessedly, laughter). We were amazed at the multiple complexities women experience when dealing with the death of an ex-husband, and so we were very happy to be creating this book in the hope of helping others who find themselves in our situation. We hope it helps you! As one of our contributors, Laurie Wimmer, so gracefully stated:

> *If we as a species are to celebrate the best in human-*
> *kind, we must be a part of making the world a better*
> *place. If we are to create beauty and love instead of*
> *poison and pain with our deeds, then there needs*
> *to be a rethinking of the treatment of ex-spouses in*
> *the aftermath of a loved one's death. We are more*

like in-laws than outlaws, but often, we are seen as inessential to the custom of mourning our dead. We may be overlooked and unnoticed or aggressively excluded, depending on the circumstances, but sometimes we suffer no less than others in the orbit of the lost spouse. Graciousness is a rare commodity here. I am sympathetic to the emotions that crowd out the ability one might otherwise have to be compassionate and thoughtful. Yet it would seem that, with a 50% divorce rate in our society, sheer humanity demands a reinvention of customs to focus on inclusiveness. If the circle of love is honored, it should be wide enough to include all who loved and were loved.

Please note: We wanted and hoped to include chapters from men who had to deal with the deaths of their ex-wives, and we did try to find them. Robyn did an online search of various discussion forums, yet all she could find regarding men's issues were discussions of financial and logistical problems resulting from the deaths of their ex-wives. If there are any men out there who would like to write about this topic from a more personal perspective, we would be happy to update this book to include their stories. We can be contacted at info@deathofanex.com and davis-floyd@austin.utexas.edu.

PART I

SURVIVING THE DEATH OF YOUR EX

Robyn Hass

CHAPTER 1
HEARING THE NEWS

I know that many people skip over book introductions. So, let me start by saying that if you only read this first paragraph and nothing else of the book, I want you to realize two important things that I hope will become etched into your mind: 1) you are not crazy for feeling the way you probably do; and 2) you are not alone.

My part of the book is much longer than the chapters written by our other contributors. It is based on the very raw journal I kept after my ex-husband died. That journal saved my sanity. At the time, I could find virtually nothing online or in print that talked about what I was going through. I came to feel alone—that surely I must be the only one experiencing such awkward feelings of grief and loss. I originally intended to make this book a single memoir based solely upon my journal, but later, I was blessed to find other women who also wanted to share their stories. I hope you will not render judgment on any of us, as our only motive is to help others who have felt lost in the grieving process by sharing the intimate truths of our lives and experiences. We don't claim to have all of the answers or the right solutions. We just hope our readers will find common ground, and know they are not alone in their grief or confusion or other experiences when dealing with the death of an ex-spouse. That said, here is my story.

Friday, December 17, 2010 was, for me, a day that started off pretty much like any other day. It was a typical Texas winter morning. The air was brisk, but not too cool. San Antonio was decorated for the holidays, and my 8-year-old son, Jarod, was wearing his best pajamas. It was the last day of school before Christmas vacation and he was pumped and ready to go. His school had planned a "fun day" full of parties and cupcakes, movies, and excitement, in preparation for the best two weeks off from school of the year.

On the way, we called Jason, my son's father and my ex-husband, as we did every morning and evening when I had Jarod. Jason honored me with the same respect when Jarod was with him. We had been separated almost two years, and divorced a little over one. Custody was split 50/50, and most of the time, my ex and I got along great, although that had changed a lot in the past few months.

We had substantial disagreements about his young girlfriend's presence in our son's life, which had recently become a major point of contention. Although our divorce was amicable, we both held a lot of pent-up anger for things that had gone wrong in our marriage. We had drifted apart over the years, and the worst part was that we saw it happening and let it keep going. I think we were both worn out by each other. I was a Type-A personality and he was not. We had gotten to the point where, even though there was a lot of love, we absolutely drove each other insane and knew we weren't right for each other.

We had met in my second year of college, when I was 19 and he was 21. Jason had just put school on hold to move home and take care of his mom, who had become ill. He was easygoing and a genuinely nice guy with a big heart. We got married about four years later, in 1999, and in 2002, I finished graduate school in a dual program in public health and social work. We planned to have our first child during school, and I soon became pregnant with our son. We both realized that because of my degrees, my capacity for income was much greater than his, so he became a stay-at-home dad and raised our son until he was old enough to go to preschool, slowly growing a web and graphic design business on the side to keep his mind from going to mush. I was enamored by his ability to care for our son and run his business. I've never seen a man have such pride, nor have so much patience with a child as he did with Jarod. He was an amazing father.

Unfortunately, the more I advanced in my career as a public health and management consultant for the Department of Defense, the more we grew apart. I stopped inviting him to after-hours office events, and he stopped asking me how my day had gone. I got sucked into the corporate world, basking my eyes on the next rung of the corporate ladder instead of the caring man I had at home. Eventually, he'd find reasons to stay up late in the home office rather than come to bed, and we found ourselves passing in the halls like strangers. It weighed on both of us. We tried a few minimal approaches to save our marriage, but the spark had dwindled and died, and neither one of us had the emotional energy to want to make it better. Resentment replaced that spark that drives a young marriage, and we soon spent little time together that didn't involve an argument.

In the November of 2008, after nine years of marriage, I told Jason I was leaving if things didn't get better. They didn't, so we rode it out through that Christmas for our family and our son, pretending everything was okay until the holidays had come and gone. In the spring of 2009, I moved into an apartment and let him keep the house. I knew the house payments were too much for him, but he insisted. He wanted to make sure Jarod stayed in a stable place he knew, despite the heavy financial burden.

In June of that year, just before our divorce was final, I met my future husband, Joseph, and Jason met a young woman who soon became his girlfriend. I was happy that he had found someone because I felt guilty that I had and was doing well. I had taken a job as a regional program manager overseeing R&D contracts, and soon after, met Joseph, who was managing large commercial construction projects.

Before I knew it, I had gone from surviving Jason's and my bankruptcy (a precursor to our divorce) to driving my boyfriend Joseph's expensive car and being able to buy my son just about anything he needed. The discontent on my ex's face grew every time I was around him. I wasn't trying to rub it in, but he was struggling financially and it made his anger at me grow. He wasn't doing well without someone pushing on him every day to get him out of his funk, as I had done for years. Jason wasn't lazy, but he had always had a hard time believing in himself and his abilities, despite the fact that he was one of the most talented graphic designers I had ever encountered. Stepping back, I realize now how depressed he was and that I missed seeing it. As a result, his business dwindled and he spent more time out at night with friends. Our initially amicable upcoming divorce turned more and more bitter. He dragged it out until I gave in and let him have most of the equity in the house. Our divorce was final on 9/9/9. To me, it could as well have been 666.

It was a horrible day. Jason didn't show up for court, which meant it was me alone asking for the judge's signature, me alone petitioning for the divorce. The whole burden felt like it fell all on me at that moment. Looking back, I just don't think he could force himself to be there, to end 14 years of us. I know he didn't want to let go of the marriage, but he didn't push very hard to save it either. I know now that we were honestly lost. We really didn't understand what true marriage was all about—two people accepting each other's brokenness and loving each other anyway because of an ultimate bigger plan. I didn't even start to learn the basics of this hard fact until years later, when a pastor's speech made my jaw drop with that, "Oh crap, he's right, why has no one ever told me this?" look on my face.

Jason was working hard, but struggling to keep up with the hefty mortgage payment. I really felt badly for him. I know he was trying his best to keep consistency in our son's life, and to save the home Jarod grew up in, but it wasn't enough. New development in the area drove up our tax rates and the payments now were just too much for any single person with a normal job to handle. I was still on the mortgage note because he hadn't been able to refinance it in his name. A year later, by the Fall of 2010, Joseph, now my fiancé, and I had to take over the house because we were receiving pre-foreclosure notices on it. That, and renegotiating the equity, didn't make things much better between us all.

Jason's and my relationship continued to deteriorate as Joseph and I moved into the house and my son became closer to Joseph. I know it had to weigh hard on Jason to watch his ex-wife's fiancé take charge of his house and help to parent his son. I felt for him, but didn't know what else to do. If we hadn't taken action on the house, we would have lost all of our equity in it to foreclosure. Jason understood and agreed. But even though he wouldn't admit it, I knew it hurt him deeply, and I hurt for him.

Our lives were changing so much in those days. For a long time, I had dreamed of leaving Corporate America to get back into the maternal and child public health field, or even to become a midwife. I missed the one-on-one interactions I had had with clients when I was in therapy sessions or leading therapeutic groups. With my fiancé's financial support, I was soon able to pursue that dream. I think this bothered Jason as well. It also meant that I was pretty much 100% dependent on Joseph's income, something Jason could never offer me despite his best attempts.

I could see how my moving forward with my life and finding happiness was eating away at my ex. I was also irate at having to take back the house, as Jason had let the maintenance get behind, and Joseph and I ended up having to put thousands of dollars into it to get it fixed up and sold. The continued turmoil over the house and my fiancé being in my son's life added to the animosity between Jason and me. I still cared about my ex, though. I don't think you can spend 14 years of your life sharing a bed, and a family, and everything in-between, and not still have some feelings for that person.

Anyway, enough about our past. Jason didn't answer the phone that Friday morning. We left a message. Sometimes he worked late, and honestly, 7:15 a.m. was early for anyone when they weren't on parent duty. The thing that really bothered me was that he hadn't answered the night before either, which was definitely not like him. He had never once missed a nighttime call with Jarod. My son shrugged it off and I dropped him off at school.

After I left the school, my anxiety and curiosity got the best of me, and I decided to drive by my ex's apartment complex to see if his car was there. It was, so I drove home thinking that he had just slept in from a late night out with his friends, or forgot to charge his phone. I kept texting and calling him, but there was no answer. I was worried and angry. He was supposed to pick Jarod up from school that afternoon for the weekend, and I had no idea if he was still planning on doing that. At 8 a.m., I started texting his friends. By 8:30 a.m., I had talked to his mom again and we were both worried. I told her also, of course, that his life was no longer any of my business, but that I would appreciate it if she could let me know if she heard from him. She asked me to do the same, and I departed for my 10 a.m. meeting downtown.

I had fallen in love with my midwifery internship. My career in public health so far had kept me in an office or only occasionally out in the field to tag along with engineers who wrote up environmental risk assessments. I longed for the direct contact with clients that my degree in Maternal and Child Public Health had prepared me for. Midwifery was a perfect fit. I got to see women in an unhurried environment, listen to their concerns, meet their families, see their growing bellies, and become a part of their lives. Nothing is more amazing in the entire world than being present when a woman musters all of the power she may not have realized she had and brings a new life into the world on her own terms. Most of the births I had the privilege of attending were home births: peaceful, quiet, and unobtrusive. It was such a stark difference from what I had experienced personally when my son was born in the hospital. I couldn't get enough of it! By this time, I had been involved in a hands-on midwifery internship for about seven months, and had been present at almost 20 births.

One of the babies we delivered that week had severe complications and was rushed by ambulance the day before (after not breathing at birth) to the hospital. I was on the phone with my preceptor learning about how great the baby was now doing. It was truly a miracle. I should have been ecstatic, but it was all overshadowed by my concern for my ex. I told my midwifery preceptor that I was worried about him and she tried to make me feel better by reminding me that he was a grown man and had probably just stayed out too late with friends and was now nursing a hangover.

While I was on the phone, my ex-mother-in-law called. I let it go to voicemail, hung up with my preceptor, and literally spent five minutes trying to fit into a tiny parking space at the retro café where I was meeting my colleague. Something in me didn't want to hear her message. Finally parked, I forced myself to listen to the voicemail. It was his mom, "Robyn, call me back immediately!" she said in a demanding, panic-stricken voice. I took a deep breath and made the call.

I don't remember the exact words she used—something like, "He shot himself"—but I do remember sitting in my car screaming "NO, NO, NO, NO, NO, NO, NO" at the top of my lungs, curled over in the driver's seat, banging my fist at the window and crying. She said she was speaking with the police. I heard her muffle the phone, tell them I was really upset, and ask if someone could come get me. I told her I would be okay, but our conversation was preempted by a deeper voice I didn't recognize. She said she was at Jason's apartment and had to hang up to speak with the police more. My heart sank into my stomach. I just sat there, alone in my car, staring out at the empty street. I was trembling and couldn't even breathe. *Oh God, how could this be happening?*

I looked over at the clock on my dashboard and realized that I was late to my appointment. I decided that if I could just not think about it for five minutes, I could go inside, explain that I had a family emergency, and leave. My colleague ended up following me outside because she said I looked pale as a ghost when I approached her. That's when I broke down in front of the large, painted café window and lost it. I barely knew this lady, and I was now flooding her shoulder with snot and tears.

She stood by while I called my fiancé. He worked in Houston during the week, building his new company, and we commuted three hours one way or the other on the weekends to maintain our relationship. I was planning to come up to Houston that weekend, but my ex had insisted that he wanted to take Jarod to his mom's for an early Christmas, so I obliged and we stayed home. In fact, he was extremely adamant about us being in town that specific weekend. Now I know why.

Joseph was shocked. He said over and over that although they didn't get along, he had never wanted anything like this to happen to my ex. He was feeling extreme guilt, even though he had nothing to do with it. I told him I needed him to stay on the phone for the 30-minute drive from downtown to my ex's apartment. He said he would, but he would have to make some calls to transition work so he could leave town, and then would call me right back.

As soon as he hung up, I called my midwifery preceptor. She was more than just my mentor; she was a very close friend. She didn't answer, so I left a voicemail, breaking into tears. At that point, I realized the scene I had begun to create in front of the tiny coffee shop window. I hugged my colleague and departed for my ex's apartment.

That was the longest 30-minute car ride of my life. I rotated between panic attacks, wanting to vomit, crying so badly I couldn't see the road, and just wanting to crawl in a hole until the horrible nightmare I was having was over. It couldn't be true. No way. Not Jason. That's all I kept thinking. *Why?*

I spoke with Joseph on the phone a few more times, stopped for gas because I was on fumes, and then spent the last 10 minutes of the drive in quiet solitude. Every time I thought of my ex, I just saw everything covered in white. I began to think of the impending funeral, and of our divorce, and started blaming it all on myself.

I sat at the light that turned onto the road to his apartment, staring at the red circular bulb and praying it wouldn't turn green. I just wanted to sit at that light all day. I wanted to hide out under it. I wanted this horrible day to be over—to never have happened! But of course, the light turned green, and the horn beep behind me forced me to make my turn.

I was now 2 minutes from his apartment. Two minutes from the reality that would change all of our lives forever. I reached into my glove box to dig for cigarettes. I hadn't smoked in a long time, but I was hoping I had left one in an old pack or something. I didn't find one—just paper oil change receipts and a flashy bejeweled cross from my Halloween costume. I ripped off the chain and stuck the cross in my jacket pocket.

I held on to it for dear life as I parked, got out of the car, and walked the steps over to his apartment.

"God give me strength. God give me strength. God give me strength," I whispered over and over again, rubbing the cross in my pocket as I got out of my car and walked through the sidewalk access gate.

When I arrived at the front steps of his apartment, I was met by a big burly police officer with his arms crossed. He looked at me with a face that made me realize he wasn't going to let me pass. I didn't want to—I just wanted to find Jason's mom, Karen. I was ushered to the next door over, a model the apartment company used to show prospective tenants. I walked up the stairs, met Karen, and collapsed into her arms, bawling.

I remember how composed she was. Upset and crying, yet composed. There was work to be done and she was strong. She and her husband, Jason's stepfather, were both there. It was awkward, to say the least. I hadn't really spoken to them much in the months that followed the breakup, except when she tried to extend her time to visit with our son. Our relationship had pretty much become non-existent after the divorce was announced. That was mostly because of me. I chose not to feed or nurture that relationship anymore. It was now weird to find myself in such a weak moment with her, but she brought something to the table I never expected. She brought grace and forgiveness, unexpected kindness and love. It blindsided me. It also comforted me and made me feel welcome when I shouldn't have been welcomed or invited at all. Then, the ultimate reality shock set in: *How will we tell Jarod?*

I about died. How could I tell my 8-year-old son that the most important person in his life was gone? My heart sank. I felt helpless. What was I supposed to do? Could I even do this? We waited for his mom's pastor to come and help us work through it all. We sat staring at the walls and ceilings and at the police walking around outside. The clock just ticked uncontrollably on the wall, like a metronome that brought you one step closer to insanity every time it moved. We just sat and breathed and cried.

The police and apartment staff came and went throughout the morning. Karen tried to distract me so I didn't see his body being carried down and wheeled away in the ambulance. I called my parents and told them something horrible had happened and they needed to come into town. They just said, "Okay," and that they were on their way. In retrospect, I know now that they knew about his death before they arrived. Looking for Jason, I had been in contact with one of his friends that morning. He had finally called me back to ask me what the hell was going on—what was so important so early in the morning? I had told him the news—and this strong, brawny, boisterous man, had fallen dead silent. After he hung up with me, he must have called my sister's husband (one of my ex's best friends since middle school), who I'm guessing, in turn, told my parents.

I called my brother-in-law's cell phone to relay the news, but my sister answered. "Is it true, Robyn? Is it really true?" she said, half-hysterical. "Yes," I responded. I don't remember the rest of the conversation, only that she was screaming and crying.

My parents arrived and I met them in the middle of the courtyard by the apartment. They were both crying. My dad squeezed the air out of me with his hug and my mom said she just couldn't believe it. Over the years, Jason had become like the son my parents never had. They had been upset with me over the separation, and not very supportive through the process. Just after we announced the planned divorce to everyone, my father made it clear that he did not agree with my decision. My family had also gotten off to a rough start with my fiancé and did not like him, which further complicated things.

My parents came up to the model apartment we were in, and like everyone else, sat there quietly, barely talking. We were all in such disbelief. Jason's mom's pastor and Jason's stepbrother arrived shortly after. I felt sick. I walked downstairs to get water for everyone from the leasing office, and stole a cigarette from his stepbrother.

When Karen's pastor arrived at the model apartment, we prayed and talked about the best way to tell Jarod. I didn't know if I had the strength to do it. We agreed that the best thing would be to tell him that his dad had an accident with a gun. We didn't want to lie to him, and hadn't been there, so without the final results of the police investigation, it was pretty much the truth as we knew it, or at least as we could spin it for an 8-year-old to understand and be able to survive. We didn't think he would come out of this even remotely okay if he knew that his dad—the man he loved more than anything or anyone—had taken his own life, and had *chosen* to walk away.

We agreed that we would all go together to Jarod's school, and that a police officer would escort us to let the school know it was serious. The school was next door to Jason's apartment, so we all went there as a group. The plan was for me and Jarod to ride with family and someone to drive my car home, but we got spread apart—every spot in the school parking lot was full because of all of the parents there to help with Christmas parties.

I drove around the semi-circle in front of the school and a lady in front of me pulled her SUV into the last slot available. My heart pounding and in tears, I pulled up beside her, rolled my window down and shouted, "Can I please have your parking space? My son's father just died." She looked mortified and hit the gas. I pulled into her spot.

I know that I took a lot of deep breaths, but to this day don't know how I made the walk inside. I kept having to tell myself, "Step, step, step, step," until I got to the door. I felt like I was going to pass out, fall over, or have a heart attack. I couldn't feel my legs and could barely catch my breath. Was I having a heart attack? "Oh God no, not me too!" I thought. "I can't do that to Jarod. Get it together!" I told myself.

When I got inside, I was met by the rest of our family, and was ushered into the counselors' offices. They had already notified the staff. The pastor suggested that everyone else wait in the conference room so Jarod wouldn't be overwhelmed. It was happening so quickly. Before I knew it, Jarod was on his way down from his classroom. I just wanted to scream, "I can't do this!!! Time out!!! Please stop this!!!" When I looked up, there was my adorable son standing in front of me in his PJs (it was "last day before Christmas break fun day" at school, remember?).

"Mom! I was in the middle of my party! Why are you here? Are you coming to my party?" God, he was so cute. I looked over and saw the entire counseling staff and most of the administrators of the school crowded together, standing in the doorway of one of the offices. Every single one of them was in tears. I had to look away or I'd start crying too.

I grabbed Jarod's hand and said I had something I needed to talk to him about. He was completely preoccupied about getting back to his classroom party, and I struggled to gain his attention. We walked into one of the counselor's offices and I shut the door. I took a deep breath, sat down, and pulled him in towards me.

"Jarod, you know I love you more than anything in the world, right?" I said. He nodded and babbled something else about his party. "I have something that is really important that I need to talk to you about, something that is really hard to talk about," I said as I pleaded and prayed silently: "Oh please, God, please don't make me do this. Don't make me take this kid's dad away from him. Please!!!"

I took one last deep breath and said, "Jarod, your dad had an accident with a gun and he died."

There was silence.

Then tears.

And more tears.

Then the questions that I don't even remember how I responded to.

He crawled into my lap, crying.

And then he asked me a question I will never forget, because it made me chuckle in the midst of the horror. "But mom, who will take care of kitty?" he asked, as his eyes filled with tears once more.

"I don't know, sweetie, but we'll figure it out," I answered with an awkward giggle.

I looked up through the slit of glass in the window and saw Pastor Scott looking in on us like a protective angel. To this day, I don't know what I would have done without him through the whole thing. I hugged my son and cried with him for what seemed like forever.

I held Jarod tight, and then told him there were a lot of people here to see him, and walked him slowly across the hall to the conference room. When I looked up, I saw that the room was filled with teaching and counseling staff, all in tears. I gave them a thankful smile, cried a few more tears and shut the door behind us in the conference room. Jarod fell into my dad's arms crying and I into Pastor Scott's.

Everyone loved on Jarod for probably a half-hour. School would be ending soon and I didn't want Jarod to be exposed to all of his friends coming out and asking what was going on. Finally, I had just had enough of the tears and sadness. It was too much. I grabbed Jarod, wrapped his heavy 8-year-old body and legs around my waist, threw open the door, and carried him out of the school. I looked back and saw that no one was behind me. I didn't care. I just kept walking.

CHAPTER 2

REALITY SETS IN

I walked for what seemed like forever to the car with my son's heavy body wrapped around my waist. My parents had this plan to drive my car so I could ride with someone, but I was flustered, and looking at Jarod, and I couldn't wait for them to update their plan or catch up with me. So I continued walking down the sidewalk, carrying him all the way to the car.

I buckled him in the back, climbed in the driver's seat, wiped the tears from my eyes and took a deep breath. "You can do this," I thought to myself. "Just suck it up and drive! It's only a few miles straight down the road. One light. Two turns. You can do this." I looked back at my son and half-smiled. "I love you so much, you know that, right?" I asked him. He nodded and put his head against the window as he stared into the street.

I drove the mile or so to our house, constantly looking back at him curled up on his seat. He wasn't crying. He wasn't asleep. He was just curled up, gazing out the window, pasty and white like I've never seen a child look before.

The next thing I knew, we were home, curled up on the sofa with him in my lap, crying. I had left the door unlocked and, one by one, the group of our family and extended family

SURVIVING THE DEATH OF YOUR EX

slowly made it through the door. I had called Jason's mom and asked her to invite the pastor back to the house. He came by for a while, but then had to go. I was almost resentful and didn't want him to leave. This was the most traumatic moment in our lives and I didn't understand how anyone could leave. I was being selfish, but in that moment, I felt I had a right to be. To this day, I am so thankful for his help and his presence.

Jason's stepbrother was really kind and went to get everyone hamburgers. It was after 3 p.m., and I hadn't eaten all day. I tried to eat a couple of French fries, but just wanted to throw them up. I was so numb. My mom begged me to eat, but I just couldn't. I was starving, but sick inside.

Joseph walked through the door a few minutes later, looking completely out-of-whack. You could tell he didn't feel comfortable in the midst of my ex-husband's family, or the situation as it had unfolded, but he did his best to be warm and comforting despite the awkwardness.

I knew that he and I needed to talk privately away from Jarod, and I desperately needed to get out of the house and away from all of the uninvited chaos. We were also really low on money from starting our new business, so I used a trip to the bank and my need for stomach medicine as an excuse to go out for a bit. I didn't want to leave Jarod, but he was having fun playing with all of the grandparents. I knew that he was in good hands, and that if I didn't have a moment away from him to simply lose it and bawl, I was going to explode.

I honestly can't remember what Joseph and I talked about in the truck on that drive. I do remember that he himself was almost in tears, telling me over and over that he never wanted anything like this to happen. I remember about halfway through calling my best friend since high school and telling her the news. At the initial request of my ex's family, I told her it was an accident (not suicide). Everyone was in shock, and they didn't want him to be remembered that way. I tried to honor their wish.

Of course, my friend wanted to know more. I finally told her the truth and we both started crying. I spoke with her for a while, and then Joseph and I made our way to the bank and Walgreens. I was in such a daze—I felt like I was in some crazy psychedelic movie, strolling the fluorescent-lit isles of the store. A part of me felt that if I could just stay there wandering the toy aisle, I could avoid the turmoil going on around me, but I knew I needed to get back to Jarod.

My son was 8, but I bought him a stuffed animal and a remote control monster truck in an attempt to help take his mind off of things. It was a week before Christmas. Everyone was officially out of school now and happily rushing around to garner their last-minute gifts. They all looked so jolly. Kids filled the isles, looking at big stockings and wondering what Santa would bring them this year.

It was as though the magic of Christmas had been sucked right out of us. Instead of planning how we were going to wrap Jarod's presents and slip them out under the tree on Christmas Eve, we were now faced with planning a funeral. It wasn't fair. No 8-year-old should have to remember Christmas interlaced with his father's death.

We returned home, and Jarod was eerily already acting like a new kid, smiling and begging Joseph to put the star on top of the tree as we walked in. We grabbed the ladder, placed the star, and then let Jarod play with his new toys. Everyone continued to alternate between hugging on Jarod and stepping out on the back patio to talk privately.

Then it seemed that just as quickly as they had arrived, everyone was gone. I looked around and we were alone. Just me, Jarod, and Joseph. The house was quiet, but eerily full of death. Everywhere I looked, I recalled old memories of Jason and of our family before the divorce.

I just wanted to get out of there. Actually, I wanted my doctor to write me a couple of prescriptions for mind-numbing valium or something to knock me out, but Joseph talked me out of it, reminding me that I needed to be there 100% for my son. He was right. Today was *not about me.*

We three made our way to the Japanese restaurant down the street. It was Jarod's favorite place to eat because they cooked everything in front of you and the chefs did neat tricks with the food. As he giggled at the chef spinning his knife in the air, I sucked back tears. How could this child be so damn happy? My therapist mind went into overdrive. I evaluated everything I was doing and finally had to realize—this was *his* grief process. This is what he could handle at this moment. He was shutting it off as a form of self-protection, and who could blame him? He had just lost the parent he loved to hang out with most in the entire world, and his fish and cat, all in one day. What did he do to deserve this? I was so angry with God. How could He let something like this happen to a child? Where was He in our grief? Our pain?

Over the course of dinner, and throughout that whole day, I went through every emotion imaginable. I missed my friend, despite what our relationship had turned into over the years. I blamed myself for his death. Maybe if I hadn't divorced him, this wouldn't have happened, I thought. Maybe if I had stayed home with Jarod and pushed Jason to have a career outside the home instead of me, *maybe* things would have been better.

I was hurt that Jason had done this to himself. I was angry and felt guilty that I was probably one of the last people to talk to him and hadn't found a way to stop him. My Type-A, over-controlling personality was pissed that he made this type of decision without consulting me, and I had zero input. I kept thinking back about the grizzled sound I heard in his voice that afternoon, the day before his death. I had known something was up, that something was just not right. I figured he was just tired and let it go. Why in the hell didn't I simply drive into the apartment complex and check on him? For goodness sake, it was a simple turn into a parking lot on the way home from Jarod's school. Even though I hadn't practiced in years, I was a trained therapist. Jason had made no threats nor even alluded to the idea of suicide, but I knew he was sad from breaking up with his girlfriend. I should have intervened. I beat myself up over that for a long time.

I felt guilty for the lost marriage. I felt guilty that he didn't reach out to me. I felt guilty that he left his son here to grow up fatherless. I blamed myself a lot, for everything. The worst part was that, in some way, I felt that everyone else blamed me too, especially with the divorce so recent. I fought back another round of tears and stared into space.

The three of us finished dinner, grabbed a few movies from the store, and headed home. I managed to get Jarod ready for bed at a decent hour, but he wanted to sleep on the sofa. I couldn't blame him. I wanted to be near him too. Word had gotten out about Jason's death and I fielded a few phone calls before crawling into bed. Everyone wanted to express their sorrow and offer to help. I hated talking about it. I just wanted to be left alone.

Then I did the most awkward thing of all—I cried and cried and cried about my ex-husband in my fiancé's arms. I'm not talking about a couple of tears and sniffs. I'm talking about bawling for hours straight, to the point where my fiancé had to ask if I had still been in love with my ex while we were together.

"Still in love with my ex? What the hell? Are you freaking kidding?" was all I could say to respond. I was furious. How in the world could I still be in love with my ex-husband? If I were, wouldn't I still be married to him? But at the same time, I had to wonder. Here I was, snuggled in my bed with my fiancé, bawling my eyes out in grief over my ex-husband's loss. What the hell was wrong with me?

We continued to talk, and I finally fell asleep in the wee hours of the morning. When I woke, I felt really good. I think I even stretched and smiled. Then it hit me like a ton of bricks falling on top of my bed and I wanted to throw up—it wasn't a dream. Jason was dead. I prayed that the nightmare was over, but really, it had just begun. I checked on my son, who was still sleeping on the sofa, and then answered more phone calls.

My sister, who had just relocated to the West Coast from Texas, called to tell me they were flying in. Her husband had been one of Jason's best friends since middle school. That's how he and my sister met—through Jason. They married a few years later.

Jason's mom called me several times that second day. They were going to start emptying the apartment. My parents came into town to watch Jarod so we could help Karen pack up his belongings. A part of me was curious as to the "crime scene," a part of me wanted to help, and another part of me knew I needed to get as much of Jarod's stuff out and over to our house as possible before it accidentally ended up in some box in her garage.

As we got into the truck to head over, I remember Joseph asking me if I really wanted to do this. He said he could just go, and help, and come back. But I insisted. There was something odd inside calling me there. Maybe it was the fact that my ex never let me in to see his place while he was alive. Maybe it was because I knew his ex-girlfriend's things were still there and I wanted to know more about the person he had told his friends had broken his heart.

I remember walking up the stairs to the apartment after the police and cleaning crew had cleared it. When we arrived, an entourage of kind souls from his mom's church were there helping. They were already busy packing up boxes and cleaning up the mess in the kitchen.

I looked over at the huge fishbowl on the bar, but there was no sign of the little Betta my son had lovingly named Sushi—only a mess of broken glass and shiny rocks strewn across the kitchen countertop and living room carpet. I dropped to my knees and crawled around the floor, looking for the fish. Jarod loved the heck out of that little fish. I knew it was dead, but I wanted to see its little dead body to be sure. No fish. At that point I realized I looked like a flipping idiot, crawling around on the floor looking for a dead fish body, and got up. It looked as though someone had hit the fishbowl and broken it. Was it Jason? Was it in his last moment of anger, frustration, and hurt before he left this planet? I sucked back tears and sniffles. No one needed me to be a drama queen. No one needed me to add to the hurt today by showing my own grief, so I hid it the best I could.

I avoided the bedroom where Jason had shot himself like the plague. Eventually, I asked Joseph to go in with Jason's mom and see what had happened. I told him I couldn't bear to go in, but needed him to see it so I could have someone to talk to in the future when I was ready to know more. He went in and helped Jason's mom understand the holes in the wall the police had dug.

Apparently, the cleaning crew the apartment hired had taken the mattress and cut out the carpet fragments with blood on them. The police had left holes in the wall searching for the bullet.

I wondered where the girlfriend was, since all of her stuff seemed to still be there. She was nowhere to be found. Crazy thoughts ran through my mind. There was a note, a small unassuming note with scribbles all over it: "Everything goes to Jarod." That was it. It didn't even look like it was in his handwriting. It was shaky. Was that all that was left of his life? A dirty apartment and a tiny note? There had to be more. There had to be something. He couldn't leave us with just that, could he?

Joseph came out and told me it wasn't that bad. Karen made a sweet attempt to cover the bullet hole in the wall so it wouldn't disturb me so much as I came in to see Jason's room and go through a few boxes. Eventually, curiosity got the best of me and I entered the bedroom. I saw the place where the bed used to be. I saw the spot where the police had dug the bullet out of the wall. I saw the patch of carpet cut out that he spilled his blood upon.

I took a deep breath and walked through the closet. I saw old boxes of things that had made us a couple: a family. Pictures. Notes. Files. Mine, his, ours. Everything was about to be packaged with all the rest of his belongings and sent out to his mom's house.

I took a deep breath and looked into the bathroom. Dried toothpaste spit filled the sink, and there was a dirty razor lying nearby. Did he shave and clean up in his last moments? What did he look like? What did he do? What was he wearing? Questions raced through my head. I took another breath and answered the call of a helper going through the stuff in the room that had been Jarod's in Jason's apartment.

It was a really cute room. Jason had never let me in the apartment to see it. When I showed him around my new place, I thought he would return the favor and show me his, but he refused and only sent pictures from his phone. It hurt, but I understood that he wanted his privacy, especially with the new live-in girlfriend. I guess I wouldn't have wanted my boyfriend's ex-wife snooping around my new place either. But it still bothered me, not knowing what my son's life was really like over there. And now here I was, going through every bit of it, deciding what to send to Jason's mom's house and what to keep for Jarod. I felt like I was betraying Jason and his wishes, intruding on his life that was no more.

Jarod had loved playing video games with his dad, so the first thing Joseph did was to unhook the Wii and pack it up for him. It was so weird being there, watching everything. Women from the church were still cleaning the disastrous food mess in the kitchen that had sat for a few days. Spaghetti. I will never forget the skillet of rotten spaghetti on the stove, or the unopened bottles of wine on the countertop that someone asked me if I wanted. I watched as the cabinets were opened for me to look for items that might have been mine.

Everything was familiar. It was his half of everything we had collected together over the course of the last 14 years. I recognized every dish, plate, and vase. All of it. And as stupid as it sounds, every piece held a memory. Watching it all being packed up and taken away was, in a way, like having something stolen. I knew it wasn't mine anymore. He had gotten those items in the divorce, but somehow, they were still ours, even though there was no longer any "us."

I helped go through Jarod's closet and picked out what I thought would fit in his small bedroom at the house. There was so much stuff; I didn't know where I was going to put it all. Since we had separated, we had each replenished Jarod's room and clothes and toys so he wouldn't have to be toting things back and forth between the two houses. The entire closet was full of board games, clothes, and Legos. There was no way we would be able to find a place for it all in his tiny room at the house.

I boxed up as much as I could and Joseph helped me carry the boxes to the car. He was so helpful. I can't even imagine how out of place he must have felt. In the course of our 18-month relationship, he and Jason had spoken on just a handful of occasions, and even then, only for a few minutes at most. It was obvious that there was friction there, as was to be expected. Joseph was now involved in my son's life, and Jason didn't like it. I don't think any loving father would have.

I went back upstairs, and as I turned the corner, the blue painted letters spelling Jarod's name hanging neatly above his bed caught my eyes. I thought about how much his dad loved him. I thought about how he tried so hard to be a good dad. Jason had always tried to make sure to spend quality time with Jarod—I can't remember a time when I ever saw Jason mad or yelling at our son. It was such a cute, well-kept room. I felt tears welling up in my eyes. I tried to escape everyone there for a few minutes, and headed outside. I completely and totally lost it half way down the stairs. I started bawling uncontrollably and sat down. A few people comforted me, but I honestly didn't want to talk. I wanted to be left alone to figure out what the hell was going on in my head. Everything I had "figured out" with the divorce, and had finally gotten my mind wrapped around, had changed profoundly. I didn't even know how all the pieces fit together anymore. I felt like the wind was just completely knocked out of me, but I knew I had to be strong for my son and for Jason's mom. Besides, I didn't feel like I had any right to grieve. I felt like every tear I shed probably just looked like an attempt to get attention. What right did I have to be sad—I gave him up, right?

One of the women from the church came up and hugged me. She told me that her son had committed suicide too and she wanted to help in any way she could. She was so kind. I felt so bad for her. I felt so out of place. He was my *ex*-husband. I didn't even know how I fit in this whole situation. I felt like a vulture going through everything to get stuff for Jarod. At the same time, I was disturbed that everyone was going through all of Jason's stuff and packing it up to send it to his mom's house, because 1) most of it still felt like it was mine because it was mostly stuff we had acquired when we were married; and 2) didn't the note say "Everything goes to Jarod?"

I about wanted to vomit. It was just *stuff*. I hated this whole thing. I felt like I was just thrown into the middle of a horrible tornado, and told to suck it up and figure it out.

How could he have done this? I couldn't believe he was gone. I was so hurt and angry that he chose to walk out of his son's life. Whether we were divorced or not, he had made a commitment long ago to help me raise this child. I was so disappointed in myself and my inability to revive our marriage. I felt like everywhere I went, I had this big red circular target on my forehead, or a big flashing sign that said, "Yep, she's the one to blame!" No one had said anything remotely like that—or even inferred it—but it was heavy on my heart. It had been less than two years since we separated, and just about 15 months since the divorce was final. I couldn't help feeling to blame.

Joseph and I helped as much as we could until the last of the larger items were loaded in the rented truck and everyone parted ways. Jason's mom and her friends were able to get a good portion of the house packed up. I don't know what we would have done without them. They were, and are, truly angels.

I went back home. Friends came over. We drank wine and beer until the wee hours of the night after Jarod went to bed. We shared stories. But I still felt judged. I still felt like the ex-wife who betrayed him. I felt that everyone still had this thought that if I hadn't divorced him, he would still be here. Deep down, I did too.

Divorce resulting from a failed marriage is a two-way street. I could outline who did what and who was more to blame, and spew out the "did you know he … ?" minutiae all day long, but I realized that we were both equally to blame.

We committed to a marriage and didn't honor it. We gave up. We listened when the world said that was okay to do and bought into it. Now he was gone, and somehow along the way, he had been turned into a freaking saint. So, in my head, if he was so perfect and wonderful, I guess they must think I was the bad guy—the reason for the divorce. I was angry.

I'm not saying Jason was a bad guy, by any means, but being the ex-wife, it's almost like people see you as the only remnant of negativity in his life, almost like you are the only reminder of bad times. Maybe they don't, but I can tell you that's the way it feels.

The days that followed are a blur. People came and went. His mom's house was full of food and cards and visitors. Nothing made its way to our house except for the food she was kind enough to repackage and bring by. My family stayed for a few days, then left. We only got one card. It was addressed to "Jarod and Jennifer" (I guess they thought that was my name).

Some of Jason's friends came by one night to tell stories and drink on the back patio after Jarod had gone to sleep. It was heartwarming to have them there, but I still felt judged. They were his friends, not mine. They had been mine when we were a couple, but not now—or at least it didn't feel that way. They had started excluding me post-divorce. It got late and I got frustrated as the visit started turning into a full-blown drunken party with my son asleep in the other room.

I finally had enough of people sizing up my fiancé, and reminded them that I didn't need to get everyone's permission to act in my life. Joseph was an amazing guy and he was going to be Jarod's stepfather, so everyone could accept it and support us or move on. I told them this was an "opt in" situation and I wasn't going to be running around begging for support. It was as if they had put Jason on such a high pedestal that they weren't sure if Joseph was going to measure up to their standards, so I had to prove his worth to them. But they forgot one thing: I didn't give a crap about what they thought. It wasn't a popularity contest. It was my life, and I was not at an age to have to ask for permission. Suddenly, everyone who hadn't been in my life by choice had stepped back in and had an opinion. I felt like I was battling on every front. In the end, they told me how much they loved Jarod and were going to be there for him every step of the way as his dad's friends, to watch over him. *I'm sure I'll make enemies by saying this, but I'll let you guess how many calls I've gotten from any of them to date to check on Jarod, or even wish him a Happy Birthday. Ask Karen how many have ever called to check on her. I've learned people are great with swift sympathy, but suck at follow-through. I'm not mad, just disappointed.*

I felt so awkward and alone. I cried off and on all the time. It was ridiculous and a tremendous strain on my relationship with my fiancé. Every night when he was home, all we talked about was Jason. I honestly don't know why Joseph still wanted to marry me.

Karen let me know that many of the bigger items in the apartment would not fit in her storage, so she was planning on donating them. My mind flashed to Jason's note; "Everything goes to Jarod." I had to honor that. If I couldn't honor the marriage, I could at least honor that. I cleared out my garage, and before I knew it, it was full of Jason's things. His friends unloaded furniture, televisions, storage bins, computer equipment, garbage, all into my garage. You couldn't even walk around in there, it was so full. It was an eerie place to be, and

I avoided it as much as I could. I kept a list and took pictures in case anyone had issues with it in probate. In the end, I sold almost every last bit of it on Craigslist, and put the money in Jarod's bank account.

I know I cried and prayed and cried a lot more as the days went on. The funeral plans began. I pushed for everything to wrap up before Christmas because I couldn't bear to do that to everyone over the holidays. I thought they all needed closure before Christmas Day so they could be free to celebrate it with their families.

Jason's mom Karen was so great to include me in the funeral planning. I know it was because I was Jarod's mom and served as his voice, but it was still so nice to be included (I know most ex-spouses are not). I helped plan as much as I could. My sister (Jason's best friend's wife) created a video that was to be shown at the memorial. We spent the days keeping ourselves occupied by scanning pictures of the past. For me, each scan turned out to be a twist of the knife, reminding me of days gone by.

The days that followed didn't get much easier. I finally had enough of the calls and wrote out a script for my sister. She was kind enough to call all of the people I had on my list to let them know of the funeral arrangements. Many had already heard through other friends, but sent their well-wishes and love. I just couldn't talk to any of them anymore. I tried to avoid everyone, but one of my dearest friends wouldn't have it. She had just returned home from a business trip and stopped by with her son, who was about the same age as Jarod. I love her for that. Jarod was able to spend an afternoon playing video games and feeling like a real kid again, instead of dealing with his dad's death and looking at old pictures. I was able to vent and share a glass of wine with someone whom I could trust with some of my most intimate feelings. She actually found a way to make me laugh in the midst of all of the despair. It was the first real sigh of relief I'd had in days.

I spent the next few days digging through more old family pictures. I didn't have all of them. Most of the more recent ones were digital and on Jason's computer. He had promised to burn me a copy of all of them as he was making copies of our home videos. Now all of that was at Jason's mom's house, being looked through by everyone. I felt so violated, like I was being raped. All of my personal, *deeply* personal and *private* family moments were now on display, and there was nothing I could do about it. If I made a big scene, I would be seen as being selfish and acting like a wench. I just bit my tongue, shut my mouth, burst into tears, and drank a glass of wine with my sister.

My sister graciously volunteered to pull all of the pictures together into a movie. She scanned and edited for days, right up until the memorial service started. We went through a lot of Jason's favorite songs, and Jarod picked the ones he liked best. It was his tribute to his dad, and we ended the movie with a note from Jarod. I was very appreciative of all of the hard work that had gone into making the movie. His old work colleagues created a few large, mounted photos of him for us to display on easels at the service. Everyone was so kind, but I was so lost. I felt like I had this permanent fakeness to me all day long, just to survive. I was the outsider, but was now thrust back inside this private world again. I had mourned the loss of our lives together after the divorce, or so I thought, and moved on. Now here I was, the ex-wife, smack dab in the middle of it all, helping with his funeral preparations.

When I approached Jarod about his dad's belongings, Jarod only asked for two things—his dad's baseball cap and the kitten. So, even though we were low on money, I didn't flinch when my sister and I took him to Hobby Lobby and he picked out a $50 glass case to put the cap in. We brought the case home, and he put the cap in there like it was the largest diamond found in the history of the world. He had such pride. This kid loved his dad like no one else on the planet, and now he was gone. How could anyone ever fill that void?

The next day, I took Jarod shopping for a suit—another expenditure we weren't in a place for, but made anyway. Jarod looked so handsome in that suit. I had always wanted to buy him a suit for the holidays or a special wedding, but it had never worked out. And now here he was, buying a suit for his dad's funeral. I fought back the tears as I asked the lady for a smaller size. Jarod didn't seem to care. He just told me to hurry up because like any typical 8-year-old boy, he didn't want to shop for clothes any more.

On the way home, I asked him if he wanted to help me pick out flowers for his dad's funeral. Surprisingly, he said yes. I found a small flower shop near our house and asked the woman if she could help us put an arrangement together. As the words, "It's for his dad's funeral" slipped out, so did the tears. I apologized in a whisper, and she just smiled kindly and asked Jarod what flowers he wanted. She was so kind and patient, working with Jarod for half an hour while he changed his mind again and again. Finally, we had our design—a handful of red flowers with a ribbon. Simple and beautiful.

The missing kitten from his dad's apartment didn't help matters. Jarod was now asking constantly about the kitten's whereabouts. I had become allergic to cats, but Jarod and his dad had always wanted one. So one of the first things they did when I moved out was go pick one out from the shelter. Jarod loved that kitten. We heard about it every time he came back home. We heard about their adventures, and how she chased after laser pen lights or climbed on the bed and purred. Knowing how much he loved the cat, I realized that my next step would be to find a long-term allergy medicine that would keep me alive while the kitten took up residence in our home. I didn't care. Whatever I had to do, I would to make him happy.

Yet, despite all of our attempts, and attempts by friends and family, the ex-girlfriend decided to disregard our requests and keep the kitten. That was devastating. My heart was broken for Jarod. Wasn't it enough to lose your dad, and then have someone keep your pet from you? I didn't understand how anyone could do that. I still don't. To this day, he still often tells us stories about his adventures with that kitten. I was finally able to help him cope with it by explaining that maybe that was all his ex-girlfriend had to remember his dad by, and maybe that's why she kept the kitten. He seemed okay with that answer.

CHAPTER 3

TIME TO SAY GOODBYE

The time finally arrived for the family's private services, which started with a prayer service at a church close to downtown. It was a turning point for me on a lot of levels. I had wanted a deeper relationship with God, but never knew how to get there. Joseph had been pushing me to take my spiritual path more seriously and reconsider my views on the church and Jesus. I had long been repulsed by organized religion, seeing it as nothing more than a get-rich scheme by preachers taking people's money. Growing up, my parents never took us to church or talked to us significantly about God. We prayed at big meals and celebrated Christmas, but it was never much deeper than that. They always told my sister and me to choose for ourselves when we got older. So in that sphere, I was completely lost.

At the first family memorial service, one of Jason's sister-in-laws grabbed me while we were standing in a group prayer. I was crying uncontrollably and couldn't stop. I didn't have any tissue left and the tears were rolling down my cheeks. She just put her arm around me and held me while a group of 20 or 30 of us prayed with the pastor. Later she told me that Jason's death was not my fault, and no one thought it was.

It was so freeing, and such a loving, caring thing to do—something I needed to hear and feel more than anyone could ever realize. Sometimes the smallest acts of kindness are the biggest things we do in someone else's life. She didn't have to even speak to me, but she did, and she changed my life that day.

Jason's mom was kind to include me in all of the family events, even though I still believed deep down that she was just respecting me as Jarod's guardian, to make decisions on his behalf and to keep me happy so they could continue to see their only grandchild. Yet I still cared about his mom, despite the divorce. I felt so guilty for the divorce, and it made me feel inadequate being around their family. I threw my ideas out here and there, but never as demands. I knew that wasn't my place.

The next evening, Joseph, Jarod, and I set off for the family viewing at the funeral home. I did not want to take Jarod to the viewing, but all of my therapist friends, as well as the funeral home therapists, said that kids who see the body actually do better in the long run. They say kids have less of a tendency to make crazy stuff up in their minds about what happened. I was mortified, fearing that Jarod would somehow see the bullet hole. Karen had let Jarod pick out his dad's favorite sofa blanket to be laid over him so he would be "comfy." I had spent many nights curled up under that ratty blanket, and now the next time I saw it, it would be covering Jason's dead body. I sure as hell didn't want to go. How was I supposed to stay strong for my son? I prayed silently for help. For rescue. For escape.

I dragged myself into the funeral home. Joseph was amazing to be there at all. I kept waiting for him to bolt out of there and say, "You know what, babe, a kid is one thing, but now a father-less kid and a dead ex-husband, and having to listen to all of his family talking about how great he was? See ya!" But he never did. As hard as it was, he just stayed by my side. He was a rock.

I walked down the hallway to find that a large number of Jason's family had already arrived. People I had loved and considered my family too, at one point, were now not just a token memory, but a memory jabbing me right in the face with hugs and sympathetic smiles. I felt so inadequate. I thought they all hated me. I thought that they all thought that it was my fault that he killed himself.

God only knows what the rumors were about the divorce. I had stayed away from his family since that time, with the exception of coordinating overnight stays for Jarod with Jason's mom, or the occasional birthday event. And now here I was, with my fiancé, at Jason's funeral. Was that tacky, bringing him? Should I have come alone? I wanted to hide. I wanted to grab Jarod up and say "screw this crap" and leave, but I didn't. I did my best to never let my son out of my sight, saying hello and hugging people as we moved through the crowd.

Eventually, we were led into a small, overcrowded room in the funeral home. I sat on the floor to give the remaining few chairs to his family. My parents and sister were there too. They looked like they had never left his family. In a way, I guess they never did. My parents still loved Jason like the son they never had, and my sister was married to his best friend. I was definitely the odd woman out.

The pastor welcomed everyone and said he wanted to ask us to share memories before the viewing began, so he could get a better feel for Jason's life before the funeral. I was completely floored. His mom and dad talked about his childhood. A few relatives interjected happy memories. Then something I did not think would happen in a million years did—the pastor looked and me and asked me to tell him how Jason and I met.

"What the hell? Are you freaking kidding me? With my fiancé sitting right here?" I looked around and realized that, thankfully, my mouth had not actually opened to say those words. I was beyond mortified. Here I was, holding my fiancé's hand, and having to tell the story of how Jason and I met, by way of a friend, tubing on the Guadalupe River. I kept it as short as I could. Every word I spoke made my fiancé more uneasy. I wanted to just melt into the floor. I was trying to be nice, but also trying to be respectful of my fiancé. Jarod ate it up.

The pastor asked me a few more questions, and I told stories of Jarod's birth and how Jason, who was 6' 4", slept on the tiny hospital sofa for ten days while Jarod was in the NICU. I'm sure I chimed in a few more times, but honestly, I don't remember. I did it for Jarod. He loved hearing everyone talk about his dad and it made him smile. I just fought back as many tears as I could, and tried not to vomit on myself. I felt that I was betraying my fiancé.

Joseph looked like he was ready to run out of the room, and I can't say I blamed him one bit. I don't think I would have had what it took to stay in that room for more than 60 seconds if the shoe had been on the other foot. But he did. And he held me. And that was the moment I realized that he was truly, fully, completely the man I wanted to spend the rest of my life with. Right there, in the middle of death's door. He loved me despite all of the chaos, and he stood there in the gap, for me and for Jarod.

Eventually the pastor wrapped up and it came time for the viewing. I dreaded that moment. What would he look like? Could I handle it? More importantly, could Jarod really handle it? I let everyone go ahead of us and told Jarod we would go when he was ready. Finally, after about 20 minutes, out of the blue, he popped up and said he wanted to go. It was almost as if this switch just clicked inside of him.

I took a deep breath, and we went in together with Jason's mom. As we walked in, his grandmother was asking Jason, "Why?" in a low tone, noticeably upset. Jason's mom quickly reminded her that Jarod was present, and asked her to stop. The rest of the room cleared a little after we entered, thanks to Karen's help. Eventually, she left too, to give us a few private moments as a "family."

I sat together with Jarod on the sofa, just staring at his dead father. Jarod burst into tears and practically crawled into my lap. With that favorite sofa blanket over him, Jason looked so peaceful. So peaceful, just as if he were asleep. I even had a moment where I wanted to just slap the crap out of my ex, and tell him to wake the hell up. But of course, I didn't.

Instead, I sat with my son and cried. I cried like I had never cried before. In silence, I told Jason I was so sorry for every-thing that had happened in our relationship. I prayed he would forgive me for all of my wrongdoings in our marriage. Then I grabbed my son even tighter and said, "Jarod, this is the last time we will all be together as a family. Is there anything you want to say to your dad?" I couldn't even see, I was crying so hard. He was crying too, for the first time in days. I took him up to his dad, covered in Jarod's favorite sofa blanket, and helped him place his hand on top of the blanket covering his dad's arm. Then I told him it was time to tell his dad goodbye. And he did. Then he cried uncontrollably and asked to leave.

I carried him out, wrapped around my waist, both of us in tears. Everyone I had ever known had come up to rescue us. I fought through the crowd and asked for a private room. The pastor grabbed a funeral home staff person who quickly opened an office for us. Pastor Scott came in to talk to us. He was so good with Jarod.

Eventually, we all calmed a bit and re-entered the family rooms. Everyone finished their conversations and made their way to the gathering that was to follow. Jason's dad was kind enough to host a dinner for everyone at a nearby hotel where he was staying. I kept out of the way as much as I could. Not by choice, but more because I was an outlier. I felt like the babysitter that had brought the kid to the party. Acknowledged, but not really part of the group. They had brought a ton of old family pictures to the gathering and spread them over a table. Jarod and his aunt and uncle (Jason's much younger half-brother and half-sister) made their way through the old pictures. I knew it was hard on everyone. I barely ate. Joseph and I sat at the back of the room closest to the door, while I kept an eye on Jarod's every movement. The evening ended on good terms, and Jarod got to see a lot of his extended family for the first time since he was little.

I knew that none of our lives would ever be the same. Jason was gone. He would never come back. That point of finality echoed deep in my soul. From the day his dad died until the day of the funeral, I had tried desperately to talk to Jarod about his dad's death. Sometimes he would ask specific questions; I avoided many of them with generalized answers because he was only 8 years old and I couldn't bear the thought of him having to deal with the fact that his dad committed suicide. I wanted Jarod to grieve, or cry, or get angry, but he didn't. Occasionally he cried, but it was rare. I had to accept that he would grieve in his own way and in his own time. That was so hard. I wanted to fix his hurt, but couldn't.

The day of the funeral finally arrived, almost a week after his dad's death. It was like watching a long video unfold in slow motion. We spent the morning picking up the flowers Jarod had created for his dad, and coordinating with family to make sure the picture movie and posters were done. A dear friend dropped off our dry cleaning.

When we arrived at the funeral home, we were ushered into a back room with Jason's family. They loved on Jarod unbelievably. I took a brief respite to walk up to the entry and place some photos and memory books on the front tables, along with some slips I had printed that reminded people to watch their conversations, because I didn't want Jarod to overhear the details of his dad's death.

I had a plan for the day and I was going to be strong. I could do this. "Suck it up and get through the day," I kept telling myself. Walking up there, I was caught by two friends who gave me long hugs, followed by a friend of the family who told me, "You were a good wife." That was just too much to handle. I thanked them, but started bawling and headed back to the family room to find Jarod and make sure he was okay. On the way back, I remember looking down at my shoes. They didn't even really match the suit I had on. It was a nice black suit from my old consulting days, yet the shoes had buckles and looked better worn with slacks. It made me feel even more inadequate when walking around. I felt completely unpolished, something that was uncharacteristic of me at events like this.

As the people flooded in, I took occasional peeks through the audio room screened-wall. Eventually, we made our way out the side door into the front row. Joseph was on my left, Jarod and Karen on my right. The ceremony was beautiful.

We had had him cremated, so it was just a memorial. There were flowers everywhere, many from people I didn't know, and the large, mounted posters of him with his family and friends that we placed up front turned out beautifully. It was a packed chapel. I had known that Jason was a kind soul, but had never known just how many lives he had touched. It was standing room only.

After all the guests walked in, I did something I had never imagined that I would do. I grabbed Jarod, planted him backwards on top of one of the reserved front pews, and told him to look at all of the people. I told him that this room, now overflowing, was full of all of the people who thought his dad was a great person and who loved him, and that was why they were there. I was hoping that maybe, when he found out someday that his dad had committed suicide and had questions about why, additional questions about whether his dad had lived a worthy life would hopefully never weigh on his mind, because he would remember seeing all these people whose lives his dad had touched.

Pastor Scott was amazing. Even his eyes filled with tears halfway through the ceremony. Jarod was called to go up front with Jason's mom to light a candle in memory of his dad. Something inside of me made me grab my phone, run up, and take a picture. I felt awkward doing it, but I also knew that one day, he might want to see it. Maybe I just wanted an excuse to go up there, since I hadn't been invited.

I cried through the whole thing. Seated between his mom and my fiancé, I held both of them with Jarod squished in between us. I looked back and saw all of my friends crying. My sister's slideshow about Jason was beautiful, even though I was admittedly hurt that, at the last minute, she had chosen to include intimate pictures of our wedding and life that I hadn't consented to. The wedding pictures caused the entire room to turn and stare at Joseph like he was an intruder. (I later created a stir over it, and my sister and I had some heated words, but looking back, I see clearly that she was just doing her best to show his life, all of it, and I love her for that.)

The service ended, and I removed Jarod as quickly as I could. I was worn out. I didn't want to talk to anyone, nor did I want him to have to relive the situation again and again in the arms of friends and strangers. We hid out in the AV room, but we were soon found by a few of my aunts and my uncle, who pushed their way through security to get to us. I was grateful for their love. I was grateful that they showed up when so many of my other aunts, uncles, and cousins didn't. I guess once you are divorced, even for a short time, people assume you are no longer attached in any way to that person. I thank God for the friends and relatives who realized that wasn't true and were there for me and Jarod, both at the funeral and in the days, weeks, and months to follow.

Joseph and I left with Jarod through a back door before everyone else and headed home. We left voicemail messages on our family's cell phones to let them know we had left, and two of my friends called to see how I was, and if I wanted company. One of the two came by with her son to play video games again. I was so appreciative to have something to take Jarod's mind off of the funeral. The other offered, but was juggling disgruntled young children. I loved them both for their kindness.

Everyone else had "plans." It hurt. My parents and sister went back to my parents' home. Jason's mom had her friends and family at her house. I understood. She had invited us, but we declined. We were all tired. Exhausted. Drained. And once again, Jarod, Joseph, and I were alone. Irrationally, I was hurt by the lack of company—we could have gone to Karen's house had we wanted to be with people. Anyway, looking back, I guess I wouldn't have known how to juggle visitors, or how to make them feel welcome.

In retrospect, I think I should have asked a few friends to help me host a small gathering at our home after the funeral. At the time, the idea of a get-together didn't even cross my mind, but going back to an empty house was almost as horrible as having to sit through the funeral service. At least at the funeral, I found myself wrapped in warmth and support. At home, it was just the three of us left to figure it out on our own.

CHAPTER 4

LIFE GOES ON ... WITHOUT YOU

Christmas came only a week after his dad's death. Before that, Jarod had decided that he wanted to spend Christmas morning at our house—the house Jason, Jarod, and I had shared prior to the divorce. I couldn't blame him. That was where he had lived for the past five years in one way or another. I wondered if that had been another weight on Jason's mind—the thought of his son with his ex-wife and her fiancé having Christmas at the house he once owned. When I had approached Jason about it, he had just surrendered the morning and said he was fine with it. I felt bad for him, and even invited him over, but he declined, saying that the four of us spending Christmas morning together would have been awkward.

Joseph went out of his way to make sure that Jarod and I both had an amazing Christmas, even though we really couldn't afford it that year with everything we had tied up in the business. Jarod really wanted Nerf guns, and after much debate, Joseph and I decided to give them to him. We were afraid that after his dad's death, the guns would cause too many bad memories, but they didn't. He loved them. Before I knew it, there were shredded wrapping papers and orange foam bullets all over the house. He needed to have a "normal" Christmas more than any of us.

I couldn't help but fake my smile. I was sad and still devastated that his dad wasn't here for this, nor would he be here for any other Christmases. We had searched through all of his belongings, but there were no presents for Jarod. The Christmas tree and ornaments were still in boxes in the garage. Jarod never asked what his dad got him. He just opened his presents from us and played happily on the floor. It made me feel even worse that this was the year his dad and I had told him the truth about Santa only a few months before his dad's death. Talk about feeling like a crappy mom!

Joseph insisted on preparing Christmas dinner, and soon, my parents and Jason's mom and stepfather—Jarod's grandparents—arrived. It was not your typical Christmas, and definitely not your typical family, but so much more full of love and thanks than you could ever imagine. Karen had somehow found time to buy us all presents. I felt horrible. I hadn't done much at all. Getting to the store to buy food for dinner only a day after the funeral was hard enough. She continued to amaze me with her kindness, courage, and grace. Somehow, having her there gave me peace. I was so grateful that they had come for Christmas.

Christmas made me a little more jolly, and I wanted to grab everyone I knew and hold them close. I returned a call from an old friend who had moved to the UK, but was currently stateside visiting her family. After she expressed her sorrow and condolences, she told me that she was deeply sorry that I wasn't mentioned in the obituary. It seemed like she was the first one who truly understood where I was in the grieving process, and how awkward it was for me. Old friends who have known you forever have a tendency to do that. Something as simple as an obituary carried with it so much unintentional hurt. It was almost like an announcement to the world to say, "You are not one of the group of friends or family, and were not officially considered part of his life."

I know that wasn't the intention, and I have never and likely will never see an obituary that says "survived by the wife, kids, siblings—and oh yeah, by the bitter ex-wife who is co-parenting his children." I'm not saying I wanted to be included in the obituary, or deserved to be, but maybe it's something our society should think about. After all, with the exception of the last year or so of his life, I knew him more intimately than anyone else in the world. I had 14 years with him. They didn't. Yes, I let that intimate relationship go, but I don't think we ever really let that person go—especially when we are still co-parenting children. They are still our partners in raising our children together, despite the judge's ruling that we are no longer an official family.

The week following Christmas was still winter vacation. Jarod and I made the best of the days off from school, yet they were nevertheless filled with sorrow and grief. Time seemed to move along without us, and I was becoming more and more depressed. Joseph had to go back to Houston to run the start-up business that basically didn't function without him, so most of the time, it was just me and Jarod. Karen called and visited often to make sure Jarod was okay, and for that, I was greatly appreciative. Everyone else went back to their lives, and I couldn't blame them. We were pretty pathetic to be around.

In the days that followed the funeral, Jarod said his room was haunted, and as crazy as it sounds, I believed him. It may sound ridiculous, but the more I find out, the more I have come to realize that there truly was a spiritual battle going on around Jason. The man who ended his life was not the man we all knew. Something dark had gotten in. I couldn't help but keep remembering the last time I saw him. He had come by the house to drop something off for Jarod. He was so disheveled: so unkempt. His eyes—God, I remember his eyes to this day—they were so empty. He looked like he hadn't showered in days, and like it took everything he had to just get in the car and drive a mile to the house to drop off stuff for Jarod. He definitely wasn't the man I had known for the last 14 years. The shaky, scribbled handwriting on his note was even more of a confirmation to us that something was incredibly off. A pharmacist friend helped us make it all make sense. There wasn't enough of anything in his system at the time of his death to cause an overdose, but the combination of pills (probably found in many medicine cabinets), coupled with his despair, was enough to send him over the edge.

With Joseph in Houston, Jarod ended up sleeping in my bed for a while. At 8, I knew he probably shouldn't, and looked up everything I could find on attachment parenting. Then I just said, "Screw it!" I really didn't need an excuse from Jarod about a haunted room to let him sleep in my bed. I needed to be close to him just as much as he needed to be close to me. I just held him, and once he fell asleep, prayed over him, watched him breathe, and thanked God for each day with him. Unbelievably, less than ten days had passed since Jason ended his life. Every day seemed like a millisecond and an eternity rolled into one. It's hard to explain. Time passes faster than you realize, but so much slower when you are waiting for the grief to end.

A few days later, I followed Karen's advice and made a trip to the Social Security offices. She had looked online and realized that Jarod could get a monthly payment as a survivor's benefit. So one morning, I gathered up all the paperwork I would need. It ended up being another stroll down memory lane that I would have preferred to avoid. I dug through boxes and found our marriage license and divorce decree. Sitting on the floor of our old house, re-reading the decree, it felt like someone standing there with a baseball bat beating the crap out of me every time I read a line that had Jason's name in it, whacking me on the head for every instance of meanness that had occurred between us, for every property division, for every bit of holiday time allotted to each parent.

I felt like such a cold wench. The truth was that our divorce had been extremely amicable. We wrote the decree ourselves and shared an attorney. We split everything down the middle. The only bone of contention was the house, which he wanted more equity on if sold, and eventually, I gave in to. I thought about the nasty letter I wrote to him when he had failed to refinance the house and the payments had gotten behind. I thought about the time I went to see an attorney behind his back when I first decided to file for the divorce—he had seen my phone records and called me on it. Most of all, I wondered how the dreams of two barely out-of-high-school kids could have turned out this way. I wondered if he would have fared better if I had never come into his life. Then finally, for the first time, I looked at the copy of the death certificate his mother had delivered to me days before. It read, "Suicide. Shot self in head."

I almost hyperventilated. This is how his death would be known for all time: *"Suicide. Shot self in head."* One day, Jarod would turn 18, get curious, and go ask for the public record— and there it would be. Then he would come and ask me why I hadn't told him the whole truth, and would hate me for it.

I stopped crying long enough to clean myself up, and eventually made it out of the house and to the government offices. I sat in line for what felt like days. I tried not to cry. I wasn't disabled—people probably wondered why I was there. Finally, I was called to a desk to determine the reason for my visit and then shuffled to another line. I sat and waited again. I thought more about his death. Was I a vulture for even being here? I felt horrible. Just when I was about to leave, my name was called and I walked to a window in the back. A kind woman was assigned to me, and by the grace of God, she worked empathetically with me to get everything processed.

She determined that Jarod would be receiving about $900 per month. I was overjoyed at the financial help, but disgusted in taking it. In the end, she told me how her life too had been touched by suicide on three separate occasions and encouraged me to find peace for the things I could not control. I burst into tears as she shared her story with me. At the conclusion of our meeting, I reached across the divided partition and hugged her before I departed—something I had never thought I would do at a Social Security office. God had sent me an angel that day, and I was so, so thankful.

Jarod's counselors, teachers, and principal had all given me their home phone numbers before we took him home that first day of Christmas vacation. I had been in contact with them a few times to let them know how he was doing, and to tell them he would be back when school started up again in January. They let me know that they would be there for him, and that any time he wanted to go downstairs to talk to the counselors, he could.

Two weeks after his dad's death, just after New Year's Day, Jarod started school again on schedule. We decided it would be best if his routine remained unchanged. School would keep his mind busy, and he did really well. Almost too well, to the point where it sends red flags up in your mind because he's not breaking down like you are, or like you think he should.

He actually came forward and asked his school counselor to help him tell his classmates that his dad had died over Christmas. It broke my heart. How could I be grieving so much while this child, who loved his dad more than anything, was telling stories about his father's death in class like it was a homework assignment? I searched for everything I could find on grief for children. I had called the children's grief center days after Jason's death, but no one had returned my call. I was hesitant to take him to a therapist without a referral, and honestly, he seemed to be coping so well, I wondered if it was something we could handle on our own.

However, his school was next door to his dad's apartment— so close you could literally see it from the playground. That meant that our drive to school forced Jarod to pass by his dad's apartment twice a day—four times a day for me. Four unbearable freaking passes by his old apartment per day, five days a week. I tried not to look over, but I couldn't help it. His apartment was in the front of the complex, so you could see it from the road. I wondered if someone else had moved in. I wondered if they would ever know what happened there. Flashbulb memories popped into and out of my thoughts. Mostly, I was just really sad, but I didn't feel like I had a right to be. I was his ex, right?

The days with Jarod at school were the hardest. I tried to help with the administrative aspects of Joseph's company, but my brain wasn't into it. Accounting fell to crap. That, and our partner was in the middle of a nasty divorce, so we had almost zero help on that front. It all piled up, but Joseph took the brunt of it. He just continued to trudge through it all—through all of my crying, through all of Jarod's outbursts, through all of the family drama—he was a rock. I wasn't. I started drinking more wine to hide my feelings while Jarod slept and while Joseph was away. I wasn't getting drunk, but a glass or two of wine a night was becoming a regular thing. It was the only thing that helped me escape from the reality of what had become my life.

No matter what I did, I just couldn't snap out of the grief. It was like a blanket over me. The worst part was that I didn't fully understand it, so it consumed me. Day in and day out, all I thought about was Jason. The good times. The bad. How I would raise my son without him. Wondering if Joseph would continue to stick around through all of the craziness. But most of all, wondering how long it would be before I would be sent away for the deep depression I had fallen into. As a trained therapist, I knew I was in over my head, but as a Type-A know-it-all, I refused to admit my weakness.

I tried to work, but I couldn't. I was obsessed with his death. I still didn't understand why he decided to take his own life. I talked to friends who worked at our bank. I talked to the police detective to question his labeling it a suicide and ask again when the autopsy results would be in. I talked to Jason's mom and his close friends. I became my own detective until his mom finally shut me down and told them to stop talking to me because it was consuming my life. I was hurt, being cut out of it, but she was right. My focus needed to be on my son, not his dead dad.

As the weeks passed, I grew tired of everyone asking how Jarod was and interjecting their suggestions for fixes, and so

I enrolled him in counseling with a colleague and friend. Yes, I should have done it out of his best interests, but I knew deep down that he would barely talk to me, let alone a complete stranger. In reality, I did it because it got everyone off my back. I did it because I could say, "Yes, he's doing better and he's in counseling," and then everyone would back the hell off. If that makes me a bad ex-therapist and a bad parent, so be it. Did he talk to my well-versed child psychologist friend? Nope, not much. But he did enjoy the games he got to play in her office. Do I blame her one bit? Nope. She was great. I thank God she had the patience to keep trying despite him constantly shutting her down. Eventually though, I did find it a bit comical to watch an 8-year-old terminate services a few months later because he had determined that he was better.

CHAPTER 5

LET HOPE ARISE

In mid-January, something inside made me decide to cut off the drinking at night and to try to get myself back in line. I set up a routine and used the monotony of administrative work for our company as a way to drown out the sadness. No one wanted to hear my pity party anymore, anyway. I was tired of it myself.

I had become the sad ex-wife with the poor kid who lost his dad. It was becoming harder and harder to remember who I was and who I had been. Going through a divorce was enough to call that all into question. His death just turned the line of reality more gray. Work was my way back out. It was concrete and real.

Then, just as things started settling into place, my periods got all wacky and I started thinking I had an ovarian cyst, or God forbid, some type of growth. I was close—Joseph and I found out that we were pregnant.

I'll never forget the day I went to see my midwifery preceptor. She was so kind. She offered the kind of midwifery and pregnancy care I wish every woman could experience. I was not really close to the gestational age of hearing my new baby's heartbeat, but she took her time and found it with the Doppler. I never heard it, but she swore she did. She even went with me to my early sonogram and convinced our backup doctor to let us play with the machine for a while so she could record it on her phone for us. I had been given an amazing gift—hope in its purest form to overcome the darkness that had saturated our lives.

Yet I still kept finding more ways to add guilt to my plate. I couldn't help thinking how an unplanned, out-of-wedlock pregnancy would go over with my family, who had already somewhat fallen away from me after Jason and I divorced. My recent commitment to Christianity had caused me to feel an even deeper guilt for having premarital sex. Joseph and I had planned to elope in December and start trying to have a child soon after, but that was put on hold after Jason's death. Not only did we feel it would be tacky to follow his funeral with our wedding, but we just didn't want to deal with either family's reaction to an elopement after his death. Plus, neither of us was in the mood for celebrating anything at that point. We were physically and emotionally exhausted.

We held off for a few more weeks and then told my son at a special dinner one night. I will never forget it. While we were outside the restaurant waiting on a table, we told him he was going to be a big brother. He got the most enormous smile on his face and literally danced around like nothing I'd ever seen, proclaiming that one of his wishes was coming true.

In that moment, I realized that God had saved me and our family in a way I could never have expected. In the midst of unplanned death came unplanned life—something we could all finally be happy and excited about, something that brought me, Joseph, and Jarod together as a family, despite all the odds. It was a glimmering sense of hope in the darkness, contained in a little ball of cells no larger than a tadpole. Being pregnant was definitely not in my plans, but it was in God's, and He rescued me in every way possible with that little + on the urine strip.

The stress of Jason's death and probate, coupled with worrying about Jarod, our fledgling business, and being pregnant at 35 did a number on my body. I was slim, but out of shape, and my anxiety was through the roof.

I finally got inspired to see a counselor for myself and soon realized why my grief had been so hard on me this time around; I had lost close relatives before, but it had never hit me for this long and this hard. The counselor helped me to see that I was dealing with so many other feelings—guilt, anger, rage, inadequacy—all rolled up and thrown into the midst of Jason's death. I soon found myself bawling in the grief counselor's office, asking her if she could even continue seeing me anymore as messed up as I was, since her specialty was *grief* counseling. Her response was brilliant: "What do you think grief counseling is?"

She helped me to realize that, as screwed up as we all are, somehow we still mostly manage to function. Yet when a traumatic event gets thrown into the midst of it all, those barely functioning balances are thrown out of whack and everything sometimes comes crumbling down. In other words, all the stuff I built up to contain the craziness of my life had just been stirred up in a giant pot, put on boil, and was about to overflow if I didn't do some heavy soul searching.

In early February, Jason's birthday arrived and the grief hit me again like a brick over the head. Jarod decided he wanted to get a cake and balloons for his dad. We said a nice prayer and he asked God to bless his dad and tell him Jarod loves him. Then he wrote a note on one of the balloons and sent it flying. He signed it with just his initials in case anyone read it later, so no one would know it was him. We took pictures and called Jason's mom, who thanked me for keeping his memory alive in such a special way. I longed desperately to do what was right. My heart, however, was still broken for my son.

Jarod really was doing really well by outside standards, but a mom knows when her son is full of crap. One day, it all came crashing down. I don't remember exactly what happened, but I had realized he was hiding his feelings more and more. He stopped talking about his dad. I finally figured out that he had stopped talking because it made me cry, and he didn't want to make his mom sad. Wow, to find out you're the reason your son has stifled his grief—yeah, talk about feeling horrible.

I just remember that Jarod finally had a huge outburst, and then just lost it on me. He was screaming and crying so hard he could barely breathe. Finally, I grabbed him and held him and wouldn't let go. I remember being in the laundry room, holding him with all of my might, and sliding down the side of the dryer until he was in my lap on the floor. He cried hysterically for what seemed like forever. I had to yell at him to make him calm down and take a breath. Then something happened. To this day, I still feel like it was divine intervention.

Out of nowhere, I started telling him a story about the tile squares. I told him how they were a like a journey. I told him that right now, we are on the sad, hurt tile squares, but over there across the room, were the happy, joyous tile squares. Then I asked him which ones he wanted to be on. He pointed to the other side of the kitchen. I asked him how he thought someone got there. He shrugged. Then we talked about all the ways you could get happy again, and that it was a journey. We talked about how it takes a lot of work and time to get to the good tile squares.

The thing I think that rang through to both of us that day was that *we should grieve his dad, but we shouldn't feel guilty to be happy again either.* I realized that was what we were both doing—feeling guilty over having any joy whatsoever because his dad was dead. I saw that guilt and grief had started to become who we were, almost like we couldn't be happy and miss his dad too. To this day, when Jarod starts slipping backwards, we still talk about which tile square he wants to be on.

The days continued to be hard and I couldn't find respite. I journaled. I prayed. I unfriended people on Facebook who didn't call or show up at the funeral. I cried. I prayed some more. Then it finally hit me that I just needed a break—from everyone, from the grief, and from this place.

Joseph and I had realized, months before Jason's death, that it wouldn't be too much longer before the growing business required us to relocate to Houston. We were blessed that things had picked up with our business, but the idea of a move had been a bone of contention between me and Jason. Months before his death, I had met secretly with a very aggressive female "bulldog" attorney who basically laughed in my face when I said I wanted to change our split arrangement and go for primary custody so we could move to Houston uncontested. In so many words, she told me to check myself and stop being selfish. She reminded me that my child was lucky to have such a great dad in his life, and that I was basically an awful person if I wanted to take that child three hours away from him and make him spend weekends in the car traveling to see him. She was right.

After that, I was more open with Jason. I tried to convince him that he would do much better in Houston jobwise. He had told me he was considering it, and, in the months before his death, I had begun sending him job links. I now doubt that he was actually considering them, but he had admitted that he would have good opportunities there, which had made me hopeful. If Jason didn't move to Houston, I was going to have to choose to live with my fiancé and new baby, or my son and raise him by myself until we could work something out with the business. I couldn't be in two places at once, and that hurt me deeply.

Now, even though not under the circumstances I had hoped for, the door for our move was wide open. Joseph was really pushing the relocation, and deep down I knew he was right. Every day when I drove Jarod to school right past my ex's apartment, I cringed inside and fought back the tears. I knew my son probably did too. The small suburb we lived in was covered in his memory—everyone had known Jason and loved him. It had begun to be too much to bear. Plus, Joseph and I were going to have a child together. But the thought of hurting Karen by moving Jarod to Houston really weighed on my mind. I was still torn.

After months of deep pondering, I knew it was the right choice. We fixed up the house, hired a real estate agent, prayed, and put it on the market in the worst economy in the history of the country. And you know what? The house sold in a few weeks for more than we expected. It was Grace.

Jason's mom knew we had put the house up for sale and was trying to be strong for us. She knew we needed to move, but didn't want to be distant from her grandson. I felt horrible. She had just lost her only son, and now was about to see her only grandchild move hours away from her.

Because of the written, but non-notarized last-minute arrangement that Jason and I had made about Joseph and me taking over the house, I didn't actually have title to the deed. Jason did. Actually, the executor of his estate controlled it—that was his mom. In our last-minute arrangement, Jason and I had agreed to basically flip the sale percentages and agreement recorded in the divorce decree (meaning that Joseph and I would get more). But his parents thought the proceeds should just be split evenly. This issue caused a lot of contention, especially since Joseph and I had sunk a ton of money into getting the house market-ready.

When this process started, I had no idea what probate was. I thought it was something that old people dealt with when they had a lot of money. Before I knew it, I was right in the middle of it all. I was thankful that Jason's mom Karen had taken over the duties of executor. Since he died without a will, everything had to be done through the courts. I hated that invasion of our privacy, but understood it at the same time. We went through the motions. She sold his car and dealt with his debts. She was amazing. I don't honestly to this day know how she did it all so gracefully under the deep loss she was feeling. We prayed a lot together in those days.

Eventually, his parents honored my revised house equity agreement with Jason, but it was a tough road. I finally had to stand up and put my foot down. It was hard. I also gained the courage to tell his mom that I wanted all of my pictures and videos back because they were so personal to me. She, of course, consented, but asked me politely to make copies, which I agreed to do. They weren't being mean by any standard—it was just hard for me to stand up for myself.

In early April, we loaded up the rented van and my car to move to Houston. Jarod's classmates had a big goodbye party for him, and I brought in treats. The next morning, Jason's mom and stepfather came to help us finish packing and see us off. It was bittersweet.

We arrived at our new house in the late afternoon and movers came to help us unload. Jarod was thrilled. He loved his new home and school. We were excited to be starting over. It felt like a huge wave had washed over us, cleansing us of the darkness we had been feeling for so long. It was new, and fresh, and so needed.

Jarod started school just a few days after we arrived. His teacher seemed great, and I had told her and his counselor in advance about what had happened as best as I could. Actually, the truth is that when I was registering him and was asked for the paperwork, I handed the registrar Jason's death certificate by accident. I was mortified. This lady had to think, "Great, we're getting troubled, whacked-out people here." She politely handed it back to me, simply saying that it wasn't Jarod's birth certificate. Of course, Type-A me said, "Sure it is—he was born in Florida so it just looks different." Then she pointed, and spelled it out to me that I was utterly wrong. The words "shot self in head" must have been blown up to 60-point font because that's all I saw as I turned beet red. If I could have just sat there banging my head against the desk in her office for about an hour, I would have.

I let them know that Jarod had been having some focus issues, but overall, was doing really well. The next day, I walked him to his classroom, where he was promptly greeted by a few dozen smiling faces. The kids and his teacher seemed to receive him well, and he looked happy enough, so I left and went home.

That afternoon, when Joseph and I picked Jarod up, he told us what a fantastic first day he had and seemed genuinely happy. I was so relieved. So, of course, nothing prepared me for the call I received that afternoon—a conference call with both his teacher and his counselor. My stomach sank and I wanted to vomit. In the nicest way, they basically told me that Jarod was acting like a very unstable child with ADHD and extreme social deficits. They said he was not obeying redirection, walking around the classroom all day, picking at his erasers, making messes, and not doing any of his work. I just sank inside.

Jarod denied it all, but deep down, I knew it was true. His teachers at his old school had felt so sorry for him that they had basically let him do whatever he wanted. How could I blame them? I had watched them cry as we told him the news of his father's death that horrible day. I knew their hearts ached for him. I could see how they could let him basically get away with whatever he wanted under the guise of his grief. But here, in this traditional classroom, that behavior was not going to be tolerated. They were kind and offered help, but the truth was that he was taking away resources from the other kids in the class, and I completely understood and appreciated their honesty.

Over the next two months, we went through a ton of ups and downs. We realized that Jarod had gone from an A student to a C/D student, but no one at his old school had graded him out as they should have. He was very behind on his math and couldn't focus on his reading. He had become defiant in class and to his teachers. As hard as it was, I had to discipline him and make him understand that while his grief was acceptable, his bad behavior was not.

We worked hard to get his grades and behavior in order, but now there was another complication in the mix. My pregnancy was not going well. In the last few weeks of his school year, I had started bleeding so badly that my midwife sent me to the ER at 11 p.m. one night. Jarod was bawling the whole time, worried that now he might lose his new brother and his mom. To make matters worse, the hospital staff and doctor were cold and condescending, and made several errors in my care. My knowledge of maternal health, and efforts to correct those errors, did not sit well with them.

In the end, I was okay, but my cervix had weakened and started to dilate—not what you want to hear at 17 weeks gestation. I was scheduled to meet with our backup obstetrician to be considered for an emergency cerclage early the next morning. We tried our best to not let Jarod know what was going on, but the looks on our faces said it all. I was not about to lose this baby, and our hope with it. I did everything I could to help reassure Jarod, but it was damning to his newly restored positive attitude. He was once again full of sadness, rage, and fear. I could imagine that all he could think about was, "Is my mom going to die too?"

It turned out that the chronic stress had gotten the better of me and had wreaked havoc on my hormones. My progesterone and estrogen levels were completely imbalanced, and so I had to go on high levels of progesterone to level them out and keep the pregnancy. More expenses we couldn't afford.

I truly felt like the world was against me. That was also the time I realized that I was the only parent my son had, and that I would do anything in the world to make sure I was alive and around to see him grow up.

CHAPTER 6

FINDING BALANCE

Around the time school was ending, about a month after we moved to Houston, we made a quick weekend trip back to San Antonio to close on the house Jason and I had owned prior to our divorce. Jarod stayed with Jason's mom for the weekend. We were uncomfortable staying there despite her invitation, and found a deal on a Holiday Inn Express down the road. It was our first night alone in months, but we were too exhausted to even go out. My bleeding had put sex out of the question, so we spent the evening talking for hours about Jason.

When Sunday morning came, I found out that the day before, Karen had taken Jarod to the cemetery to see his dad's resting place for the first time, without us. I had never felt rage like that in my life. She had promised to wait until we could all go together. Talk about every feeling of being a momma bear trying to protect her young coming out! I was so freaking angry that I wanted to explode. But what did I do? I questioned it politely, bit my tongue, and said we would be out shortly to pick him up. I hung up the phone, and started screaming, crying uncontrollably, and hitting my rented hotel pillow. I felt so betrayed by her, and so unable to protect my little boy.

Over the hours that followed, Joseph helped me gain my composure and come to an interim peace with the situation.

We picked up Jarod and politely parted ways back to Houston. I stewed over it for weeks until I finally got the courage to ask her not to do it again. We again found healing, but it was hard. I had to realize that it was her loss too, and Jarod was the closest thing she had to Jason. I learned to stop being so over-controlling and quick to anger. She was deeply apologetic. In the end, it wasn't worth fighting about. I guess I was just hurt because I wanted to share that moment at the cemetery with Jarod. I was his mom, and I wasn't there for it. I felt like I had failed him again.

Over the summer, I enrolled Jarod in a few day camps to keep his mind off of things. I think it was also to keep me on a schedule. It guaranteed I had to wake up early, get dressed, and get him off to camp by 8 a.m. It also gave me time to focus on our business during the day, and my growing belly. We had found an amazing midwife in Houston and having kid-free, alone-time to see her for my regular checkups was also a much needed girly respite.

The six-month mark and Father's Day arrived in the midst of it all. I took Jarod to the store to get Joseph a gift, and as usual, he picked out a typical boy-bathroom-farting type of card. I was hoping he would one day be able to let Joseph in and to love him as a close stepfather. But for now, the cards with butt jokes were a good start. Once he picked a card for Joseph, I pulled him aside on another row, bent down and asked what he wanted to do for his dad. He said he just wanted to get a card for his dad's grave. Tears filled my eyes in the middle of the store, as well as the eyes of the lady I didn't realize was standing near us on the aisle. I wiped my eyes and told Jarod that I loved him, and that I was so proud of how brave he was. He wasn't sad, just very matter-of-fact. He picked out the card and we left.

When we got home, he wrote out the card and stuck it in the mail to Karen. She was kind and put it in a Ziploc bag and then took it to his gravestone. She even took a picture to show Jarod that it was there. He looked sad, but was okay. I learned over time that the heaviest weight on my son's shoulders was not losing his father, but worry over whether his dad was in a good place. It was consistent. Jarod always prayed on his dad's birthday, on Father's Day, and at Christmas for God to take care of his dad, and for his dad to be in a good place.

The summer following his dad's death was literally one of the hottest on record in Texas. Our small company had grown tremendously, and I was now on partial bedrest, in and out of the office as much as I could be, training my replacement before my maternity leave. Six weeks before my due date, I decided out of the blue to sit down one day to make a list of all the passwords and procedures. I had no idea why I chose that day, but sure enough, as soon as I got home, I started feeling like my pants were too tight. Less than five hours later, I was delivering our son and watching him slip into the NICU as a 34-week-old preemie.

Looking back, I realize that I had been dehydrated, and had become overly stressed about the business and insufficient capital. The topper: that afternoon was Jarod's first day to ride the bus and he got off at the wrong stop, which sent me into a panic, literally running down the street, looking for him in the 100+ degree Texas heat and two-inch clog heels. Stupid, stupid, stupid.

Having a premature labor was scary enough for Joseph and me, but for Jarod, it was terrifying. I had chosen to have a natural birth and he could literally hear me screaming down the hallway. I was blessed to have friends he knew come and watch him, but I had no idea until later about the fear of loss that he was coping with in those hours. Not only was he scared that I was going to die, and he would have no parents, but also that he might lose the baby brother he had been praying over since the day he found out about him. Thank God neither came true.

Our new baby, Jacob, was such an amazing addition to our family. As our midwife said with teary eyes, he truly unified us as a family. Now we were all related. Jacob has never, and will never be called the "half-brother." He is a gift that inspired us all to open our hearts and realize that we were still capable of loving deeply after such a series of tremendous tragedies and tests of our faith.

School started up in the fall, and soon it was winter again. Jarod was faring much better than before, but was still having focus and concentration issues. He said he worried about everything, and his teachers said he spoke of Jacob constantly.

Like most blended families, we struggle with what it is to be a family. From my perspective, I do believe that we struggle much more deeply than most. Joseph finally came out to really share how he felt during those months following Jason's death. He said that he initially felt guilty for the role he had taken over in our lives, and guilty that he wasn't always overtly friendly to Jason when he was around. Most of all, he said he that he had felt trapped after the initial shock of Jason's death wore off. Jarod was still Jason's son. Joseph was the "other guy," who all of a sudden became the only father figure in Jarod's young life. Joseph said he felt like it was all thrust upon him overnight, and no one stopped to ask him how he felt about it.

Of course, I didn't know any of this for almost 18 months after Jason's death. Joseph could have turned and run on many occasions. I think a lot of men would have. Jason's suicide was a lot for anyone to deal with, but I can't even imagine what Joseph had to go through when it came to things like the looks he got at the funeral, or all of the awkward family moments that followed. In retrospect, it helps me to understand all of the minor arguments we got into when we moved to Houston. They weren't really about the stupid stuff we were fighting over; they were about dealing with roles being redefined overnight, and not having a way to push a "pause button" to try to cope with them. We were always moving forward, and because of the day-to-day circumstances in our lives, we never had a free moment to stop and take it all in. I realize now that I really didn't give Joseph the emotional distance he probably needed to sort it all out because he was the one person in the world I bared my heart and soul to, day-in and day-out. If I had given him a break from my needs at that time, I know for sure that I would have fallen apart.

I realize it sounds selfish, but I have to say that it's sad how few people really step in to support you as the ex after the funeral is over. I was lucky to have a ton of great friends and family, yet most of them stopped following up on us all after a few weeks. I'm not mad about it. I understand. Life goes on. Joseph was my rock, but in the process, I forgot that he needed a break—needed time to breathe—and most of all, needed a chance to make a decision to be a father to Jarod, rather than have it just assumed that he would be.

Thanksgiving soon arrived and we headed back to San Antonio for a family meal with Jason's mom. Jarod stayed with her, and we stayed in a hotel so that everyone wouldn't have to endure 3-month-old Baby Jake's 2 a.m. and 5 a.m. feedings. It was a nice, relaxed Thanksgiving. We let Jarod stay at Karen's house until Saturday morning.

That is a morning I will never forget. We arrived to pick up Jarod, and he came at me with rage and anger. His eyes were full of tears. When I asked him what was wrong, he growled "You know," clenched his fists, hit the bed, and fought back the tears rolling down his face. I tried to console him and talk to him, but he wouldn't have it. He was angrier than I had ever seen him. He would only say, "Nana told me and you already know." Finally, she walked into the room and I forcefully demanded, "What did you tell him?"

In her kind, ever-so-polite voice, she told me that she had talked to him about some of the prescription drugs she found in his dad's room when he died and that they caused him to make a bad choice, and that's why he died. I literally felt Jarod's rage come over me. I wanted to yell every curse word I knew at her. I wanted to spit fire. I had never been so mad and hurt and angry in my life. This was MY child. It wasn't her place. I was so red, I must have turned white on every extremity of my body from the lack of blood flow to anything but my face and chest. Outside of the room, she told me that Jarod had been prodding her and wanted to know. Jarod later denied it.

I could barely breathe and have no idea how I held it all together to get my crying, hurt son out of the guest bedroom, packed, and in the truck. To this day, it is still a blur. I can't believe I kept my composure until we got on the road. Then I lost it. All the way home, while Jarod just lay in the back-seat, upset. It was like someone had stolen his heart—the last broken remnant of it had just been ripped away. I was so angry and hurt that I could barely get my words out to Joseph. It was one of the longest car rides of my life. I didn't want to dig for details. Did he now know his dad killed himself? I couldn't dig. I had to let it go. What was done was done. I know Karen didn't have the intent to hurt Jarod. I know she was trying to help him work though his grief, but she wasn't living with him every day. She didn't know where he was at. It took a while for me to work up the nerve to talk with her about it, and she agreed to redirect those conversations to me from now on. I know she never intended to hurt him. Jarod was shaken, but later seemed okay. I walked away, believing that he really didn't get the concept of suicide from their conversation, and life once again moved along.

The year anniversary of Jason's death snuck up on us. His mom had decided to have a small memorial service at his graveside. We weren't in a position to travel, and I frankly needed a break from his death. Jarod didn't want to go, so we didn't attend. I quietly put the word out to all of his friends and my friends, but sadly, none made it there. She saved some of the flowers and the prayer for me to give to Jarod one day.

I was really disturbed that it had already been a year since Jason's death. I looked out at the full moon. It was not much different from the huge blood moon that circled our house the night after his death. I felt like I was living it all over again and had to push it inside to not deal with it. It was Baby Jacob's first Christmas, and I was determined that it would be a good one for all of us. This year, we celebrated alone in our new house and let Jarod Skype with his family across the country. It was small and intimate, and just what we all needed.

Jason's birthday rolled around again in early February, but this year, Jarod didn't want to celebrate it. I honored his wishes and helped him call his grandmother. I still felt so bad for her losing her only son. I wanted Jarod to somehow want to remember and honor his dad, but I didn't want to bring him back to the level of grief he had been facing in the past. I knew everyone had their own timetable, but I also soon realized that I was imposing mine on Jarod, thinking that if I was still sad, surely he had to be too. He was sad, but he also wanted to start living his life again, and for that, I was truly thankful.

In talking to others who had lost parents, I realized that a big factor in the continued grieving was the empty spot at the kitchen table—something we didn't have to experience. I'm not saying that Joseph replaced Jarod's dad, but he did bring a masculine presence and structure to our home that I think helped Jarod move forward, or at least cope day to day.

At the time, I didn't understand whether or not Jarod had fully grasped what he had been told by Jason's mom that Thanksgiving weekend. Only about six months later, when I got pulled aside by his new Sunday school teacher (yes, "Welcome to the new church, we need to talk!") did I realize that Jarod actually understood that his dad had chosen to take his own life. The teacher (also the head of the children's ministry) pulled me aside to let me know that when the children were drawing things that represent how good can come out of bad, Jarod had asked if it was okay if he drew his dad committing suicide, and then draw a picture of his little brother. Can you hear my screeching mental tires?

Holy $*$&%(*&#*$&*!

So picture this: it's 14 months after your ex-husband's death and you finally feel like you are getting your life back together. Out of the blue, you get pulled aside after church service in a busy hallway to get told about your son's morbid drawings, and asked if there is anything the new church you just started going to can do to help. Can you say "cry me a river of freaking tears" right there in front of everyone? I was beyond mortified, and of course, it was a full service, so a bazillion people passed by us in the hall on the way to get their kids. The worst part was that I had bottled everything up inside for so long, the damn tears wouldn't stop flowing. As soon as they did, she would say something nice or give me a hug, and there they were again. Stupid tears. Of course there was no bathroom to escape to without another long walk to the front, so I just gave up and made my way with my family to the car.

We talked about it in the car, and Jarod was really okay with it. I had no idea that he even knew what the word suicide meant. He did. He explained it well. He said dad took drugs and he wasn't himself, and life got to be too much for him to handle so he shot himself. Well $#**###$$***##!. Yep, I guess that about says it. I guess now I have one less thing he will hate me for when he turns 18 and decides to move out.

Karen and I have since worked it out, and set boundaries about what she will and won't talk to him about. I think she was just in a place where she was truly trying to help him understand better and absolutely meant no harm or to overstep her bounds as a grandparent. I love her and totally forgive her, because in the end, I think it wound up being a much better way for Jarod to learn about his dad than becoming 18, pulling the police records, and calling me a lying you-know-what.

In late April of 2012, a little more than 16 months after Jason's death, Joseph and I were finally officially married. We decided to have a private ceremony with only a few friends, and to rent a beach house for the weekend. It not only saved us a lot of money, but also a lot of drama. No one can truly understand your life and the choices you make except you. While these chapters tell our story, they leave out a lot of ancillary drama surrounding our business and daily lives that I just didn't feel up to sharing—days that were nothing short of a bad reality TV series. I can say honestly though, those few years were, by far, the most excruciating and overwhelming time of my entire life, and to this day, I don't know how I actually survived.

We sent out dozens of wedding announcements, but only received cards or quick emails or comments on Facebook from a few people. I have a large extended family, and their lack of response was hurtful. I concluded that they were either busy, blamed me for Jason's death, or just didn't care. I cried it off and kept moving forward. I had an amazing man in my life who loved me, two wonderful children, fantastic friends, and a relationship with Jason's mom that made me feel like I had a functional family again. The rest didn't matter.

Over the months that followed Jason's death, Karen and I became much closer. I think we both realized how short life is, and that love and forgiveness were more important than anything else. We supported each other spiritually as well, which made a huge difference in both of our lives. I'm sure we still get on each other's nerves from time to time, but ours is a relationship I wouldn't trade for anything. I love her and her husband dearly, and they have even taken Jacob in as their own grandchild.

I know it has been more than an awkward road for Joseph to travel—welcoming your wife's ex-husband's family into your new one so fully. He has been truly gracious and open about the entire situation. As a result, we have all gained tremendously. It may not be your typical family, but it is the most genuine love, and I am deeply grateful to have Jason's mom and stepdad in our lives, as is Joseph. God filled our hearts and lives so deeply, and we are profoundly thankful. Sometimes, in the midst of tragedy, if you can find a way to open your heart, you can have opportunities to find deeper, more meaningful relationships and amazing love in the oddest of places.

In May, Jarod finished third grade. He was doing much better, but was still struggling with attention issues, and his grades had been suffering as a result of missing key math facts that he should have learned the year before. We worked hard at picking up the missing pieces, and this time, he walked away with As and Bs.

Father's Day weekend marked 18 months since Jason's passing. This year was different. Jarod said he didn't want to talk about it or do anything for his dad because it just made him sad, and he wanted to move forward. He bought Joseph another funny fart card, signed Jacob's name on it, and we had a small Father's Day celebration at the house. I wanted him to do something for his dad, but I realized that was my need wanting to be fulfilled, not his. Baby steps.

It took me a long time to see that since just after the funeral, Jarod has been cautious of his feelings around me. He is very protective of me and realized early on that his dad's death made me sad, so he held back for a long time because he said he didn't want to make me cry again. We worked through those feelings, and I became more and more able to talk about his dad's death without crying. Now, however, he was holding up the white flag and saying, "Mom, I need a break from it all." I understood that completely. We all need a break from time to time. No one should have to live in grief forever. He had a right to be happy and move on with his life.

He asked me to put away all of his dad's stuff and stick it in his closet. It was just a few pictures and some photo albums. I asked him to reconsider, but he was adamant. He said he couldn't focus on his homework because it distracted him. I agreed to put it away if he promised not to bottle up his feelings about his dad. He pinky swore and then said, "Mom, really, I'm good."

Over the summer, I realized that I wasn't in need of one-on-one counseling anymore, but still had a need to talk about Jason's death. I decided to attend a Survivors of Suicide group. Joseph was kind enough to rush home early from a long day so that I could go. There were about ten people in the room—all very welcoming. One of the leaders had lost her son about a decade ago, and the other was a therapist there to guide the group. The entire group was really supportive and asked me to speak about Jason's death.

I thought it would be great to get it out, but when I finally started talking, I started bawling and at times, could barely even talk. I realized how mad at him I am for leaving Jarod. I realized how much I hated him for having to deal with everything on my own. I recalled how much it sucked going through the funeral. I also realized that I probably didn't fit into the group.

As we were wrapping up, they passed around a stone that you were supposed to hold and say a message to the person you lost. I wanted to say, "You're a selfish a-hole," or "How the hell could you dump your kid and walk away without even telling him goodbye or leaving a will?" but I refrained. I started crying and said, "Jarod missed you for his birthday and Father's Day," and passed the stone along. There was a part of me that hated them for making me say anything at all.

I walked out with a few of the ladies, who were awesome, and I promised to come back. But I didn't. I just couldn't bring myself to sit in a room full of people who were sad about losing close loved ones when I wasn't. I missed Jason as my friend, but by now, I had more anger and hurt than grief. It wasn't fair to them. Sure, I missed him as my co-parent, but it had been a long time since I was in love with him.

The tears come far less these days for both me and Jarod, although he does still have occasional meltdowns that I think are the result of being overwhelmed on a lot of levels, and also not knowing how to handle life as a kid without a dad. Joseph has been a great shoulder, but he will never be able to replace the innocent love that was destroyed when Jason took his own life.

I still think about Jason pretty much every day for one reason or another. It can be something as simple as wanting to call and share one of Jarod's accomplishments with him, or just being sad that Jarod can't build a Lego tower with him. This week, it was because Jarod had a primary role in the school play, and Jason wasn't there to see him perform. I can't tell you what it's like to be so proud of your child, and then fight back tears in the middle of a huge group of fellow moms. I guess it made me realize that you never know what someone else is going through and shouldn't pass judgment.

Sometimes I accidentally come across old photos in my computer and think about the past. There is a naiveté lost in divorce that I don't think you can ever really find again. Whether you realize it or not, a part of your innocence is cut out with those pen strokes and judge's ruling. When you compound that experience with the death of an ex-spouse, I think it is amplified extensively. So is the hurt.

You don't really have the open opportunity to be angry with your ex anymore. You can't make pithy comments about things they do that drive you crazy to keep you from going crazy sad over the divorce. As horrible as it sounds, I think anger can provide some balance that keeps you from mourning too heavily. That person with whom you shared the births of your children and the most intimate details of your life is not there anymore. That co-parent, partner, and friend is gone, and you will never have the chance for reconciliation. That person who is supposed to be there for your children regardless of the divorce—a tie that is supposed to never be broken—is no more.

In essence, I think that when the anger that overshadows a divorce is replaced with hurt, and emptiness, and death, the unresolved grief that has built up about the divorce finally rolls in along with the grief of the death like a bad monster storm that has been off the coast, picking up wind speed. You're hit out of the blue with this huge gust and totally weren't expecting it. It knocks you over. That's what it did with me. It took me a long time to realize what was going on and to move forward, from grief—to anger—to forgiveness.

I think surviving the death of an ex is not a one-time thing. It's a journey. It transforms you, and if you find a good path, you might even find it takes you to places of healing and hope that you might never have found. At least that's what it did for me.

When I was finishing my chapters for this book, I asked Joseph if he remembered ways that I coped. I thought his answer was perfect. He said, "You didn't cope. You lived. You kept going day by day because you had to. You never really found a way to cope—you just held on because you knew that each day, it might get a little easier until it was bearable." So true.

Sure, I'm still sad over Jason's death, and Jarod's and Karen's resulting loss. Sure, I'm still angry that he left us. But at the same time, his death reminds me each day how precious life is, and how little we really know about the lives of the people around us and what they might be going through.

His death made me live a little less aggressively and a lot more peacefully. The biggest place I had to find forgiveness was in the most unexpected place. I had to learn to forgive myself and walk away from people who wouldn't let me. I had to put my family above drama, and I had to fight daily for my son's heart before it slipped away to an overdose of hurt. When I look back one day, I might find that the decisions I made to protect my family may be disapproved by many, but I would make those decisions over again any day, despite how hard they were, and still are.

Twenty-three months have now passed since Jason's death. Looking over at the living room tonight, watching Joseph and Jarod laughing and playing on the floor with little Jacob fills my heart with a joy and peace I never thought I would feel again. Our life isn't perfect, but it's off to a good start.

This year, we spent Thanksgiving at Jason's mom's house again. This time, her annual celebration included her husband's children and his ex-wife among the 20 or so people attending. What a wonderful model for what a family can be! What would life be like if we all just got over ourselves and our egos and found a way to make a family work—exes included—no matter how disjointed and chaotic and crazy we may find that? What if we all finally realized that being an ex doesn't mean you are no longer part of the family?

I guess what I'm saying is that by the grace of God, I found a remarkable path to healing and peace in the most unthinkable place—with my ex-husband's family—and we are all stronger in so many ways because of it. They have opened their hearts to accept and include Joseph, and Karen was even kind enough to write a letter to be included in this book. I've decided to keep most of it to myself, but will share with you the last part. I am still in awe of her strength and ability to love so deeply through all we have been through. She wrote:

> *Having walked the path of loss many times before, my eyes were open to the "emotions" that could have turned this tragic event in another direction. I am forever grateful to God that [Robyn's] heart was soft and that her fiancé is a spiritual man also with compassion and a desire to support her and my grandson through this loss.*
>
> *I know that, for both the former wife and the parents of her former husband, being single-minded in our desire for the child from that union to feel loved and for that child to know that both are compassionate and caring of the other is the key. What we all gain is "family." Our memories of happier times are the same and we can share them still and pass them on to this precious child*

*who is the best from both of them. And, we have
the opportunity to make new memories and bless
each other throughout life and life's many twists
and turns. Truly God does restore 2 fold what the
enemy has stolen, Isaiah 61:1-9"*

After Thanksgiving, on the way home, I asked Joseph to
take us to the cemetery. He stayed in the car with Jake while
I took Jarod over to his dad's grave. We sat and talked for a
while. I won't share all of the details, but I will tell you that I
still have to fight like crazy for my son's heart so it doesn't slip
away to hurt and anger. He bottles a lot up. He blames God.
He blames me—maybe things would have been different if we
hadn't divorced. He's right—maybe they would have been. But
none of us will ever know. We just work on it all day by day.
We struggle for healing and fight like crazy to build the bonds
that grow and strengthen families.

It was surreal, visiting Jason's grave for the first time. I
take comfort from my sense that his soul is at peace, but I still
miss my friend and co-parent. I always will.

I wanted to write my part of this book to share our story.
Our pain. Our hurt. Our confusion. My feelings of being totally
and completely lost and alone, and the joy we all managed
to find on the other side of tragedy and loss. In the end, I
wanted someone going through the loss of an ex to have what
I didn't have—a story that called out and said, "You are not
alone." But no matter where I went, I couldn't find another
soul who would come forward to share a similar story. Surely,
other divorcees had been through the same thing, but they
were silent. All I wanted to hear was, "I've been through that.
You're not crazy. What you're feeling is not weird, and you'll

get through this. I promise. Be strong and have faith." But I couldn't find it.

I hope you will find it in this book—in our compilation of stories from me and from others who have been there. Believe it or not, you will get through this, and you'll probably be stronger at the end of the road. You might even find that the road will take you to better places than you could have ever expected.

I have found a deep peace on this journey that I never thought possible—peace with my ex, with our former relationship, and with his untimely death. I'm definitely not perfect, and four years later, I still sometimes find myself crying over the whole situation as my son grows into a teenager without his father. I thank God for Joseph—that he stepped forward with an open heart and helped fill a void that is so often left empty. Life is still rocky and bumpy and uncomfortable, but the good days have finally started to outnumber the bad. Time really does help heal our wounds, and I hope that yours heal sooner rather than later. Above all, though, I hope and pray that you are able to open your heart and find forgiveness and that deep, deep peace that grabs hold of you and doesn't let go.

PART II

Survivors' Stories

CHAPTER 7

ON BEING AN EX-WIFE WHEN YOUR EX-HUSBAND DIES: WHAT IS YOUR SPACE? WHERE IS YOUR PLACE?

~ ROBBIE DAVIS-FLOYD ~

I was on an airplane in Brazil when I got THE CALL. The plane was close to departure and the flight attendants were about to tell us to turn our cellphones off. Mine rang, and I saw that my son was calling and figured it must be important (he almost never calls when he knows I am traveling), so I answered.

> And his voice, full of tears and pain, said: "Mom, we lost Dad today."
>
> Me (I'm thinking, *lost* him? Did he wander off somewhere?): "What? Can you please say that again?"
>
> Jason, speaking very slowly and clearly through his tears: "Mom... we... lost... Dad... today."
>
> Me, screaming now: "Jason, are you telling me that Robert died, that he is *dead*???"
>
> Jason, sobbing: "Yes, Mom, he died, he is dead."

Me sobbing louder: "What? HOW???"

Jason: "He died in his sleep—Debbie found him this morning, just a few hours ago. He was still warm, but not breathing, so she called EMS, but he was already dead."

Me, trying to catch up to my shock and to sort the thoughts racing through my head—I was on a research/fieldwork trip to Brazil that Robert had funded—how to honor his memory best?—should I continue with the trip to honor his funding of it, and his clear desire for me to complete it, or should I race home, leaving my colleague and friend, Nia Georges, alone to continue with the rest of the trip, and conduct the remaining interviews, and cancel my already-paid-for flights and scheduled talks in the next two cities of our six-city trip? Two seconds to think it through, and then the answer comes clear in my mind; *"I have to go home to be with our family and to support my son!"*

Me: "Jason, I'm coming home. I will be there as soon as I can! This plane is about to take off. I can't get off it, but I will arrange in the next city to take the fastest flight home."

Then the plane did take off, and I was sobbing in Nia's arms. She held me tight all the way from Curitiba to Brasilia, where we were supposed to change planes to go to Recife to conduct more interviews with Brazil's amazing holistic obstetricians—our current and very exciting anthropological research project, and where I had promised to do an all-day workshop for the birth-activist community there. And I was thinking, "Robert is dead. He's only 63—how can he be dead? He can't possibly be dead! I love him so much—he has been my supporter and benefactor, and one of my dearest friends. How can I possibly live without him? How can Jason, his son, who totally adored him? And Debbie, his wife—she will be more than heartbroken—and their daughter Erin, age 10. Oh, my God, she is going to have to live the rest of her life without her father!! I lost my father at age 23, and it took me ten years to recover. She's only 10!"

On the tarmac in Brasilia, during our transport from one tiny plane to another, in my broken combination of Spanish and Portuguese, and still in total shock, I managed to convey to the runway guys that my "husband" had died (I couldn't think of how to say "ex-husband" in Portuguese, and they didn't understand my Spanish—*mi esposo se murió*—so I cut my hand across my throat and acted dead—that worked!), that I was not going to Recife, and that I needed my suitcase. I hugged Nia goodbye, trying to think about what she would need from me to complete the trip—oh right, she was out of Brazilian cash and her bank card wasn't working, so I gave her all of my Brazilian *reales*, and promised her that I would email everyone and ask them to receive her in the same way they would have received me. Still sobbing, I was ushered into the airport, and some minutes later, my suitcase miraculously appeared. Those runway guys were so kind!

Suitcase in hand, I rushed to the American Airlines counter, only to find that it had closed for the evening and would not reopen until 8 a.m. Lucky me, to be stuck in a Brazilian city where I had friends! With shaking fingers, I called my friend Rodolfo Gomez, but the number didn't work. Hanging on by a thread, I called my other dear friend, Daphne Rattner, who got me in touch with Rodo, who gave me his address and offered to come pick me up. No need; I took a taxi to his condo complex, where he met me at the front entrance. He, too, held me while I cried.

Safely settled in his comfy apartment and fed dinner by Rodo and his lovely wife, I got online as soon as I could, immediately discovering an email from Robert's wife, Debbie, asking me to write his obituary. The word hit me like a brick. His *obituary*? Are you sure he died? Shock can really make you nutty.

Determined to do the job assigned to me, I took my computer to the beautiful park, complete with streams, pools, playgrounds, and lots of night lights, that forms the center of this condo complex deep in the heart of Brasilia. I tried, very hard, to talk to Robert, to channel him to help me write his obit. Nothing. So I accessed myself, my love for him, my understanding of who he was and what he believed in, the gorgeous obituary that he had written for our daughter, Peyton (still on my laptop), and the beautiful moon above, and I managed to write the first draft of the obituary and send it off to Debbie and Jason. I sat there, sobbing, until Debbie wrote back that it was beautiful, it was perfect, she loved it, "Thank you so much!" A contribution—I had made a contribution!

Arriving home the next day, I went straight to Debbie's house. My son, Jason, and my daughter-in-law, Ashley, were there, plus Debbie's whole family and lots of other people. Debbie took me into the master bedroom where Robert had died, and spent some blessed time with me to tell me how it all happened—how she had fallen asleep with their daughter, Erin, gotten up in the morning, and gone into the bedroom she and Robert shared, noticed that he was not snoring as usual, went to check, found him not breathing, but still warm, started CPR, tried to call EMS, but the cell wouldn't work in the bedroom, had to stop CPR to go into another room where the cell would work, called Jason and EMS simultaneously so that Jason would hear her telling the paramedics that his Dad was not breathing. Jason was instantly in his car and on his way over. The medics went first to the wrong house, finally arrived at Debbie's house, intubated Robert and took him away, trying to save him, but he was already dead. As Debbie spoke, I could almost see Erin drowsily walking down the hall toward the bedroom in her PJs, asking her Mom, "Why are all these people in our house?" and Debbie telling her, "Daddy is not breathing. They are trying to help. They are taking him to the hospital."

So that was my precious hour with my ex's wife, during which she caught me up on events and made me feel included. All of my sympathy and empathy were with her, her daughter Erin, and my son. Debbie's mother and sisters served dinner. Afterwards, Alan (my significant other at the time, who had also stopped the international trip he was on to come straight home after receiving my news) and I went to Jason and Ashley's house, where we spent a cozy family evening decorating their Christmas tree and hanging out with their baby, Jax (my beyond-adorable grandson), because we all cumulatively got it that *life goes on.*

Well, life indeed went on, but the planning of events following Robert's death went on without me. In the following days, Debbie's house seemed to always be full of people getting the autopsy results (Robert died of a massive heart attack—his heart had swollen to twice its normal size), making plans, arranging the progression of events—a process I had fully expected to be part of, yet I was simply not invited. Instead of coming home to what I thought would be a hurried organizing of a Memorial Service with all of us helping, I found that Deb and Jason had decided to postpone that event in order to plan it with time and forethought. All they were planning at present was a simple viewing for "family only" (that did, thank goodness, include me). Robert hadn't wanted a viewing, but Debbie and Jason did—"selfishly," they said—but I didn't think it was selfish of them to want to see him again one last time. I did too! They knew he wouldn't want a regular fancy casket; he hated caskets in general, and he wanted to be cremated, so Robert's brother Jim, working the Internet at Debbie's house along with Jason, found an Austin carpenter who would build a simple, architectural pine casket (Robert was an architect), and we did have that family viewing at the funeral home. Deb and Jason chose to dress Robert's body in the clothes he typically wore: blue jeans, blue denim button-down long-sleeved shirt over a black T-shirt, his UT baseball cap, and his prescription sunglasses.

When I entered the viewing room alone and saw him like that, I was struck by the fact that he looked incredibly normal, and fully expected him to just get up and walk out of there. I completely lost it, sobbing like a baby, and there, suddenly, was Ashley, holding me and loving me to get me through. I did feel part of things at that moment and was grateful. But later, when Deb was in there with her husband's body, I went in to join her, hoping to have some kind of "co-wife" moment in which we could, for just a few seconds, share our grief. I tentatively approached. Just as I realized that Deb was talking to Robert with her hand on his heart, and I should just *get out*, she turned, saw me, and ran out of the room, mumbling "I will talk to him later." My bad! And so much for shared grieving—clearly not happening. A huge loss for me, added to by a huge sense of guilt for inappropriately invading their space.

After the viewing, Robert's brother, sister-in-law, their children and grandchildren, Jason, Alan, and I spent a few hours at Waterloo Ice House telling funny stories about Robert and generally reminiscing—that was a sweet time in which I did very much feel included. Deb and Erin had chosen to go home, and Ash had to take Baby Jax home, so they were not there to share that sweetness.

That was pretty much it for me as the ex in terms of any kind of inclusion in any kind of process around Robert's death. I had honestly thought that we all were part of a family—the Floyd Family. I guess I thought that because after Robert's and my daughter, Peyton, died in a sudden, terrible car wreck in 2000, Robert, Debbie, and I did everything together. For starters, we planned and put on Peyton's Memorial Service together (with the help of many other loving family members and friends). In the ensuing months of unbearable pain, Robert and Debbie came to my house on so many nights to check on me, be with me, hold me while I sobbed, and tuck me into bed when I was exhausted enough to sleep. There was the Easter dinner at a restaurant when Debbie said she had forgotten her cellphone and didn't mind because "Everyone I care about and might need to call is right here!" And there were the years when they all came to my home on December 23 for our family Christmas dinner, and many other holidays and events celebrated together. I honestly believed that we all (Robert, Debbie, their daughter, Erin, Robert's brother and sister-in-law and their kids and cousins, and of course my son, Jason, and his wife, Ashley) constituted an extended family.

Then, so very suddenly for me, it became obvious that we did not.

Debbie cancelled our Christmas evening together—she told Jason to tell me that she and Erin were not coming. I was devastated—in my mind, it was a *family tradition*. So I called her and left a voicemail saying, "Okay, you are not coming, so could Alan and I come over on Christmas Day to bring our presents?" and I got an email from Debbie in return: "Please respect our privacy. My whole focus right now is on Erin, and you are not part of her grieving process. Please do not come over on Christmas Day."

Well, I was already in enormous pain over losing Robert. Yes, he was my ex, yet he was also the *great love of my life*. We had been married for 20 years, raised two amazing children together, and enjoyed many happy times and special moments. We became incompatible over time; he hated my career, which entailed my leaving home for short, but frequent periods of time, and I resented him for hating the career that I loved. There was pain and emotional abuse; I could write reams about that, but find that I really don't want to go there. Eventually, we divorced. Yet I never stopped loving him, nor did he stop loving me. Debra was a much better wife to him than I ever was, or could be, yet our love continued; he showed it to me through ongoing financial support, and we showed it to each other in many phone and email conversations. Some months before he died, I emailed him that sometimes I just wanted to hear his voice, and he emailed back, "My voice will always be there for you."

So yes, we were divorced, yet he remained, in many ways, the bedrock, the foundation of my existence, and my sense of safety and support in the world. Then he died, so very suddenly and unexpectedly, at 63! The bedrock dissolved into dust.

I had *no one* to support me in my grieving process. Excluded and banished from Deb's house, where everyone always seemed to be gathering, I grieved alone in my own home, crying on long winter nights for hours on the floor pillows in front of the fire. Alan had to leave on business for three whole weeks less than a month after Robert died. Ashley and Jason were busy with their own lives, and their baby, and often seemed to be hanging out with Debbie, who didn't want me anywhere around. Even when Alan came home, he did not support me at all as I grieved Robert. This kind and caring man, whom I had met a couple of years after Peyton died, had been nothing but supportive of my ongoing grief over my daughter, but he simply could not understand why I was in such sorrow over a man who had often been cruel to me, and whom I had chosen to divorce. He would walk by, look down at me crying on the floor, shake his head, and walk on. I didn't blame him—I found it confusing myself! I laid on those pillows for two or so hours almost every night for over two months while the tears poured, and thousands of memories flowed through my mind: the happy times raising children together, our long driving trip all over Mexico with me giving him Spanish lessons in the car, our always soul-satisfying lovemaking, the fights, the periodic drunken abuse, the many mistakes we both made in our relationship—my anger over his mistakes, my guilt over mine, the endless wondering—would we, could we have stayed married if I hadn't screwed up so badly, so many times? *Was* it my fault, as he had so often said?

In fact, I was in such pain, and so confused about it, and felt so alone, that I sometimes had a strong desire to take all the sleeping pills in my cabinet. Knowing that you should call someone for help when you are thinking those kinds of thoughts, I went through my list of friends, and realized that all of them would be asleep. Who could I always call at 3 a.m. when I had a problem? Robert!

But Robert was dead. I did try, sobbing in front of the fire, to call on him, but I never got an answer. No cosmic message, no sense of his presence—so unlike when our daughter, Peyton, had died, yet came to me many times in dreams and visions over the course of years. So those first months after he died were pure hell for me. I could not find any space or place to share mutual grief. I have seldom felt so very alone.

Deb and Jason spent a great deal of time planning the Memorial Celebration for Robert. Not a funeral—he had already been cremated—but a Life Celebration. I wanted to help, but I was totally excluded from the planning process—they had it well in hand, and did not need or want anything from me. That was devastating. My mother raised me to be a born and bred hostess, yet there was no way for me to be that now. No contributions that I could make, nothing at all for me to do.

When someone you love dies, it helps—it helps a lot—to have something to do! After my father died in 1973, my mother and I planned his funeral together. After my mother died in 1995, I planned her funeral with help from others. I've already mentioned that after my daughter died in 2000, Robert, Debbie, Jason, and I planned and carried out her Memorial Service together. I wanted, needed, to *do something* about Robert's death, something for him and the family, yet there was no role for me, and therefore nowhere to go with my grief. I have to repeat—it was devastating, lonely, and very, very hard. Of course, it was harder for Deb and Jason, as their loss was so much greater, yet they had people around them all the time (or so at least it seemed to me). I admit that in my loneliness and grief, I was jealous of the support they had when I had none.

Finally, weeks later, the invitation to Robert's Memorial Celebration came via email. Deb and Jason had planned a huge party in Robert's honor. I (mistakenly, as it turned out) assumed that Robert's Memorial would be open to any and all, as regular funerals usually are. So, moving instinctively into my hostess role, I forwarded the invitation to a few people whom I thought Deb and Jason might have missed, only get a reprimand from my son: "Mom, the venue we found has limited space. We invited everyone on Dad's cellphone list. There is no space for more people. You can't invite anyone else!"

Again, I felt shut out. I had inadvertently created a major problem—I had forwarded the invitation to my best friend, Rima, and she was planning to come. I knew that Robert, my ex, had resented Rima for many years, for really stupid reasons that had to do with things that happened in the mid-1980s— Rima and I were both part of a spiritual group that eventually became a cult, and as soon as it did, Rima got out, and three months later I did the same—yet Robert always and forever blamed Rima for getting me involved in the first place.

I thought/assumed/trusted that a Memorial Celebration would be an appropriate opportunity for reconciliation, yet Jason chose to honor his father's wishes, and thus exclude my best friend. I saw that as perpetuating the poison. I had a fight with Jason and Ashley about it via text messaging—they are Millennials and that's how they mostly communicate. During that fight, they repeatedly told me, "It's not about you!" Ouch, as in major, major OUCH—because so obviously, none of it, not one single bit of it, had anything at all to do with me in spite of our 20 years of marriage, the two children we had raised, and the fact that we had still cared deeply for each other. Of course I capitulated, and they won, and my best friend did not attend the Memorial, to deep regret on both our parts.[1]

At the end of the text fight, after Jason and Ash had clearly expressed to me how much undue stress I had caused them, I found the words to explain how hard it was to find "my place and my space in our mutual grieving of Robert." Ashley texted back that my space and my place were all about supporting Jason. Just to put an end to the whole issue, I wrote back, "Got it!" Yet *it wasn't true.* Jason had already made it clear that he did not need my support in any way—he had plenty of support from Ashley, his friends, and the extended family of which it was clear that I was no longer a part. Terrible, simply terrible for me because I was an only child who spent many hours of my younger years watching *The Waltons* on TV while crying and begging God for siblings. Loneliness cast a long shadow over my childhood, and I had so hoped during my adulthood to bask in the light of an extended family. Nevertheless, I had to accept that there was really no space or place for me and my grief within what I thought had been our family circle. It all was so very clearly *not about me.*

I wrote Jason and Ashley a letter of apology for having caused the problem and its ensuing stress on them. They did not respond for over a week. Jason is my only remaining child,

---

1   I am happy to say that after Robert's Memorial, Jason and Ashley chose to let go of Robert's negative views about Rima, and to love her for the loving, kind, and generous person she is.

and my relationship with him and his wife, Ashley, my adored daughter-in-law, means absolutely everything to me. So that week of silence, combined with my grief over losing Robert, which brought up all over again my ongoing grief over losing our daughter, Peyton, and my ongoing feelings of confusion and guilt about the failure of our marriage, plus my aloneness at home—well, you can perhaps understand that I had suicidal thoughts. I had learned by then that such thoughts need not be acted upon, but must be acknowledged and even honored as expressions of profound sorrow and despair. I had developed a deep understanding that suicide is an inherently selfish act. It might have gotten *me* out of my pain, but it would have caused a whole lot more pain for my son to lose his only remaining parent. So I just stuck it out through the nights of sobbing on the floor by the fire.

Blessedly, my co-mother-in-law Connie (Ashley's mom) helped a lot. I finally called her to try to understand why Ashley hadn't responded to my letter of apology; it turned out that Ash had been out of town at her best friend's bachelorette party. In an act of love and compassion for me, Connie let Ash know that I was in pain, and Ashley finally wrote me back, accepting my apology and getting us back on track together. *Huge relief!*

The relevant point here is that I couldn't find any place for myself in what I had thought would be a *family* grieving process. According to an article I recently read, "Place is a pause in movement, a source of nurture, a haven of stability, and a container for meaning"[2]—precisely what I could not

---

2   I use this beautiful quote with deep apologies to its author—I cannot find the article in which I read it so I am unable to provide an appropriate citation. If anyone reading this book knows where I found it, please email me at davis-floyd@austin.utexas.edu

find in the process of grieving my ex. Yet I did ultimately find it—though only for one day—when, nearly three months after Robert died, the Memorial Celebration that Debbie and Jason spent so much time planning actually happened. Explaining that Celebration needs a bit of context.

Peyton died on Sept. 12, 2000—four days before her 21st birthday. We figured out quite quickly that we did not want to have a funeral for her, but rather a celebration of her life, and that it had to happen on her actual birthday, Sept. 16, to take the place of the birthday party she had been planning to have here in Austin with family and friends. So within four days, Robert, Debbie, and I—with lots of help from many others— put together a Memorial Service/Birthday Party for Peyton at Umlauf Sculpture Garden in Austin. Over 400 people came. Our son, Jason, served as Master of Ceremonies, first speaking on his own about his relationship with his sister and telling lots of funny stories, then orchestrating the sequence of people speaking about Peyton and the huge impact she had had on their lives, followed by her friends playing guitar and singing songs for her. Then we served a catered dinner based on the menu she had cooked herself for her graduation from Natural Gourmet Cookery School in New York City, complete with a full bar. People formed groups on the lawn, moving chairs to share their meal together and talk a lot. We gave plenty of time! Then, a birthday cake lit for her 21st birthday— carrot cake, her favorite—champagne, and everyone singing "Happy Birthday" to Peyton. To this day, everyone who was there will tell you that it was the very best party they have ever attended![3]

---

3   For a complete description of Peyton's Memorial Service/Birthday Party as an example of a "ritual that worked," please see The Power of Ritual by Robbie Davis-Floyd and Charles Laughlin, Daily Grail Press, 2016.

With Peyton's gorgeous Memorial as precedent, Jason and Debbie decided to have an equally marvelous celebration of Robert's life. The venue they chose, after searching all over Austin, was the magnificent Commodore Perry Estate—lovely graceful buildings and a huge, beautiful lawn. Robert loved music, so they had a Big Band playing as the guests arrived, with our local upcoming Cat Edmonson as lead singer. Then a service on the lawn, during which selected friends spoke eloquently about Robert and the meaning of his life to them. We all learned things about him that we had never known! My son, Jason, age 28, was Master of Ceremonies, as he had been at Peyton's Memorial when he was only 16.

Searching for the right place to sit, I noticed that the entire Floyd family was seated to the left of the podium, but the seats to the right were unoccupied, so I chose chairs for Alan and me almost in front of the podium, yet on the unoccupied right side. I finally felt that I had found my place. I was right there in front of Jason when he spoke, and was heart-warmed by the several times he acknowledged me as his mother without making a big deal of it. He simply noted that his face was getting red in the sunlight because "I have my mother's complexion," nodding at me and smiling, and in introducing his godfather, Phillip, he noted that Phillip had been there at Jason's home birth, and had helped Robert to build the "womb room," complete with hot tub, again nodding and smiling and gesturing at me as the mother who had given him birth. I glowed.

Of course, he also acknowledged Robert's wife, Debbie, in multiple ways, for their happy relationship of over a decade, for their daughter/his sister, Erin, and for Debbie's planning of this beautiful event.

The feeling that I had at last found my space and my place was massively reinforced by the many people whom Robert and I had known together during the 20 years of our marriage who sought me out to greet me, hug me, and express their ongoing love and concern for me. One of them actually said, "You know, he never stopped loving you," and I found tremendous healing in that acknowledgment of what I had always known to be true. We couldn't live together—we were simply incompatible. Debbie was a much, much better wife to him that I ever could be, yet our love never died and never will. I think, believe, and hope our love now constitutes a universal energy force that will be forever ongoing, and I find a great deal of comfort in that hope.

I am an ex-wife grieving my ex-husband's death outside of the family context that others share. Yet for that one night, I did find my space and my place, and that finding continues to carry me.

Epilogue: My Quest to Forgive

I was planning to stop on that happy note, but upon re-reading Robyn's eloquent and honest chapters in Part 1, which describe so graphically her struggles to come to peace with the failure of her marriage and the death of her ex, I felt that I owed our readers a bit more information about my own struggles toward that same end. Remember those winter nights I spent sobbing on the floor in front of the fire in the months after Robert died, and how Alan would just shake his head and walk on by? One night, he stopped, stood in front of me, folded his arms across his chest, looked down at me, and asked in true puzzlement, "Why are you spending so much time crying over a man who tortured you?" I guess I must have been ready to get up off that floor, because his words hit me like a thunderbolt, and I thought, "Why, indeed?" And I did get up, and abandoned grief for anger, sometimes even rage—I spent a lot of ensuing months being very, very angry at my ex for the very many times he was mean, cruel, sometimes even vicious to me. I remembered how, during the last months we had lived together, I had promised myself that I would do everything I could to save this marriage that was clearly falling apart, and how I had tried, every day, day after day, to love Robert more, and show that love more clearly, to be the wife he wanted, only to be rebuffed again, and again, and again until that one more rebuff—one probably just like all the other ones—had become the straw that broke the camel's back. Something had snapped inside me, and clarity had descended—*this could not go on*—it was time to let go, time to get that divorce. We had, and we had both moved on, and now he was dead, and I was furious at him for, oh, so many reasons!

I can see now how that anger helped me to deal with his death. I guess I unconsciously used it as a replacement for the grief that had been consuming me, because it was impossible to feel *nothing* about him—so if not sorrow, then rage was what I had to feel. I hung out in a very angry space for quite some months after the Memorial, and the self-righteous part of me kind of liked it there.

Yet I had watched a very close and dear friend die from a rage against her ex-husband so deep and all-consuming that it turned into several different types of cancers that literally ate her alive from the inside, and so I knew that this too had to pass; I had to find a way to forgive Robert for all the hurt and pain he had caused me, and also to forgive myself for all the hurt and pain I had caused him.

I started with old family pictures, in order to bring back the good memories, the happy times. I talked with a therapist and with a lot of close friends. I had long, profound conversations with my daughter-in-law, Ashley—she really wanted to understand what had happened in the marriage that created her husband, and so she asked a lot of insightful questions that took me deep into introspection. Her careful, open-hearted listening and refusal to judge helped me express pain I had been hiding, see truths I had been avoiding, and cry tears that needed to flow. (Not only did these conversations help me in my forgiveness quest, but they also helped to generate the marvelous relationship that Ashley and I now share.) Finally, I got on a plane to the East Coast to visit one of Robert's very best friends in the world, Dave Freeman—a man in his 80s whose wisdom, I hoped, would give me the final piece of the puzzle of how to forgive and find that peace that Robyn speaks of at the end of Part 1. I wanted to see Robert through Dave's eyes, to know what he thought made Robert the great and generous and brilliant man he was, and how that great, generous, brilliant man could also be the man who had caused me so much suffering and so thoroughly wrecked my self-esteem during the last ten years of our marriage.

It was a trip well worth taking. Over dinner, David explained Robert to me in ways that I had never understood him before. I won't repeat everything he said, but I will say that he nailed it. He told me that Robert was a man whose greatness was a result of his weakness, a man so driven by his own insecurities and childhood neuroses from repeated parental abandonment that he covered them up with a charismatic personality and a conviction that he was always right. Dave said that Robert's apparent self-security and self-confidence made him both charming and fascinating, while at the same time, serving to cover up his deep feelings of inadequacy. He told me that nothing I did or didn't do could ever have made our marriage work because I was a strong, independent woman committed to a career that Robert both admired and resented—resented, because every trip I took to speak at a conference or university triggered his childhood abandonment issues. In other words, he emotionally experienced my leaving as *abandonment,* and reacted by hurting me back. The small, abandoned boy inside of Robert could not have acted in any other way than lashing out at me; our marriage could not have survived. David saw Robert in all his goodness and in all his weakness, loved him for all of it, and helped me to do the same. During that dinner, the last jagged jigsaw piece of my forgiveness puzzle nestled gently into place with a tiny, final mental "click!" I flew home with forgiveness in my heart, for Robert and for me.

—and for Debbie. I had harbored no anger nor resentment towards her, yet I had, as I've expressed above, felt hurt by what I perceived to be her exclusion of me from the family circle I thought we both formed part of. Now, with the benefit of hindsight and David's wisdom, I can see that there was no right or wrong about it—Debbie's and my definitions of family were simply different. She followed her heart and her instincts in the choices she made, as I must follow mine.

Now, I find that I can celebrate the love Robert and I shared, find release instead of pain in my grief, and live in that peace true understanding brings. Yes, guilt still plagues me sometimes, angry thoughts still surface, and resentments still simmer, but they don't boil over; they just kind of melt away because I *get* that Robert couldn't help himself be better to me any more than I could make myself into the wife he really needed, the wife Debbie became. She is a strong, independent career woman too, yet she during their courtship and after their marriage, she chose to work together with Robert—something I couldn't do because I'm an academic with no head for business. And she never left—she was always there, both with him and for him—so their marriage worked where ours could not.

Yet Robert and I conceived, birthed, and raised two marvelous children together, we loved, and laughed, and cried, we had tons of fantastic adventures, and too many fights—*it was what it was*, and that is enough. My place now is in the family constituted by my son, my daughter-in-law, and my grandchildren, and in the career that I could not abandon to make Robert happy without completely losing myself. My space is the planet Earth, which I travel as part of that career, taking my love for my family, including my ex, along with me wherever I go.

CHAPTER 8

PRESENCE OF AN ABSENCE

~ KIRSTEN DEHNER ~

I thought it would be easy. I was so sure I had a solid picture of the story I'd be telling. I should have been afraid. The first words I put down about my ex-husband's death were not what I expected. What unspooled across my page described the house where I now live, in Mexico. I couldn't imagine what it had to do with Bob's death 13 years ago. To be so clueless about the obvious was reason enough to fear. My house is filled with things he bought, most of them without me. Some sat in storage for decades; only now, in my new home, can they be seen again. Thirty-three years after our divorce, I realized for the first time, Bob is here. He's been here all along and I hadn't noticed.

A nearly eight-foot-high theater poster titled, *Moorish Illusionary Fantasy, Le Danse Des Passions*, has pride of place in my living room and dictates the wall color. I have no idea where Bob found it, or what he paid. A dark blue sky set between the arches of an Arabian palace escapes the poster frame to wrap its twilight around my living room. In the print, an Arab prince twists a dark-haired dancer's wrist as a British officer is held back, trying to defend her. Women in burkas and bearded men in turbans ring the scene. This emblematic image of colonial strife and domination testifies to the ugliness that continues to flow from that defining era. Who knows if Bob made this connection when he purchased the late 19th century piece, but he had a thing for the magic of images, and he had strong political views. Oddly enough, the region's troubled history marks the end of our relationship as well, because Bob died twelve days after 9/11. I wish I had been with him when he bought it. I don't know where he got the two stained glass windows either, which I took out of their wooden frames and put together to make a coffee table. The stories of these things moving through hands and spaces may be hidden, but their silent past, and his, informs my living room.

If I sit on the couch with the table in front of me where the poster rises to the ceiling behind my head, I can see, out of the tall many-paned windows across the room, a mesquite tree crowned with feathery leaves. I wake up every morning to the chatter of birds in its branches. Yesterday, I found bits of eggshell on my flagstone patio beneath the jacaranda that, just weeks ago, drooped cascades of purple flowers. The house is mine for the moment; I have clear title to the building and the land. But when I think about the trees and the nesting birds, my title means nothing, of course. The birds and trees belong to each other, not to me. Which brings up the next set of unexpected questions: to what and to whom do I belong, and have I ever belonged? Who am I? Who was Bob, and who were we to each other?

I call Bob's things his because they don't feel like mine. I inherited them, as is true of the Victorian drop leaf table purchased by my mother that sits in one corner of the living room. When I die, *Illusionary Fantasy* will hang on another wall, and my night room will lose the reason for its color. But the room doesn't belong to me, either, does it? It belongs to time, to the now invisible hand of the woman who built it in rambling progression over nine years. She pondered its dimensions, its entrances and exits, worried over the money, and paid the workers. The rooms I've altered in this house? I can agree that one room speaks mostly of me, and the rest we share, until someone else makes her mark, or the place turns to dust. How strange to be a child of time, to know what I feel is mine will pass into other hands, the familiar spaces and their contents altered or disappeared into the flux of memory. It has been said that the human experience of time is an illusion. If this is true, can it also be true my very personhood is an illusion as well?

Ed Ruscha's *Mocha Standard Station* print hangs above my second couch; it was a birthday present from the 60s, also from Bob. He brought it home one afternoon, a January surprise. It was shortly off the press when it passed into my hands. Bob knew Ed Ruscha, and our sons played together for a while when they were little. Danna, Ed's wife, and her Frenchy and my Josh live on as vague figures in a sandbox at a park in L.A., where we once sat and talked while watching our boys, now middle-aged, in this slippery, sideways thing I call my life. Danna, always a lovely presence, had long dark hair and dressed in great style, but she, too, has dissolved into a near void of wavering images. My son, Josh, coming in clearer now, sits on my lap in his OshKosh overalls, his upturned face a kiss away, the chains on the swings a vertical blur. Upstairs, near the window that looks out upon the mesquite tree's trembling green, a tape of Josh's first sentences sits in a drawer, his little boy's chirping voice as surely vanished as his father's, though our son lives.

The large milk-glass school globes that softly light my downstairs also come from Bob. Seven of them are scattered across my living room, bedroom, bathroom, and kitchen. More divorce booty from Los Angeles. Stacked in a tall cardboard box and wrapped in newspapers along with their fixtures, they were shipped from L.A. to New York in 1981, shuffled from one storage bin to another. After my second marriage ended, they threaded the cordilleras of the Sierra Madres, arriving here in 2008, where I finally installed them in my remodeled house in 2010. Unbroken after 30-plus years, his lights light up my home.

I got tired of talking about Bob in this way. Here's the last sentence before I quit; "Upstairs is one piece Bob and I picked up together in Minneapolis in 1965, soon after we were married: an old oak ice chest with fancy brass door hinges. Beautiful. Was he beautiful?" This is another question I didn't understand at first. Bob obsessed over the beauty of images and the stories they could tell; it was his work. Yet I often got the feeling that he didn't see a similar story in himself. Did he want to secure an image that made him feel handsome, as if being an attractive man wasn't enough? I'd catch him glancing at himself in the mirror on our downstairs landing, or in some restaurant reflection, or in whatever passing mirror gave him that opportunity. I can't say for sure what he was looking for, but I can pretty much guess it was something he could never find there, and I can pretty much guarantee that he didn't know how to look for it anywhere else. To me, those glances felt like pleas, like longings for an elusive self he wished were beautiful, but wasn't. What do I know? This could be made-up nonsense, more about me than him. What I do know is that this aching vulnerability was tied to a sweetness that touched me from the beginning. Which is why, on our second date, I reached across the car to touch his face, and that began. What?

I changed my approach to a "Dear Bob" letter, hoping I might find value in trying to find fresh ways to tell him I love him. However, this only generated more scary questions like, "Did I ever, and do I now, love Bob Abel, father of our two children, film director of rock-and-roll and other documentaries, visual effects pioneer and mentor to many, seven years older than I?" For an emotionally abused child, love can be a feeling that's hard to identify.

Childhood photos show Bob playing WWII soldiers and cowboys. There's even one of him sitting on the toilet. When it was trotted out to show me, he found it embarrassing. As embarrassing as I felt when my father burst into my bath one day, laughing as he took photos of me naked and pre-pubescent, only to post them in the family album? My father's energy was so weird, it made me uncomfortable. Why charge in uninvited, and then laugh while snapping photos? It raised a question I was too young to ask, and couldn't answer for the longest time; is my body mine or his? I know now he laughed because he was doing me wrong, knew it, and couldn't help himself. But that was typical, wasn't it, for him to be unconscious, and for me to feel absent, as if I didn't belong to myself, but to others?

Here is where I began to wonder if I'd slipped down the rabbit hole. I could feel myself spinning and falling backwards into the dark recesses of a forgotten, or even unknowable self. I'd thought that addressing Bob might open the door to unexpressed feelings between us, but it turns out that the Technicolor feelings are all about *me*. Odd that early on, we both felt compromised by a voyeuristic eye. How might this play out in our story? Did we share a common drive to repair unpleasant childhood images? When I was fighting for custody of my children, not wanting Bob to have the chance to deliver what I was sure would be his inevitable neglect, we were both subjected to psychiatric review. My lawyer never showed me the report, but said the shrinks felt Bob and I were very much alike. I think I could stand to see that report now.

But Bob Abel is gone. What does it matter whether we were alike or not? What matters about any of it? Bob's light now shimmers in the memory of those who knew and loved him, in the work he left behind, and on pages where his legacy is talked about, though less and less as time passes. His work feels more solidly present than he ever did. *Elvis on Tour, Let the Good Times Roll, Mad Dogs and Englishmen,* several David Wolper documentaries, visual effects commercials that garnered him countless Clios, *Star Trek, Tron,* two big IBM projects, one of them in the Library of Congress, on and on. In a class I once attended, the Nobel poet Derek Walcott scribbled on a blackboard the answer to a question about why writers write: *immortality.* I wonder if Bob was aiming for the same thing. Sometimes our work survives nature's drive for dissolution, but mostly what persists is our DNA splitting time on the chromosomal spirals of our progeny.

What makes us real to ourselves when we're alive? Bob has disappeared under a cloak of dissolving images where nothing is and everything once was. He often spoke of the "presence of an absence," a phrase he picked up from one of his shrinks that seemed to resonate for him. Certainly, he was absent in our marriage in ways that helped to end it, but then, when I think about absence, I have to consider mine. Maybe it's my own absence that is all I can speak of with any fidelity.

I don't know why, but when Bob's sister asked if I wanted to view his body a day before his memorial service, I said no. It wasn't squeamishness. I'd watched both my father and mother die. My father said goodbye in a way only he could: sending us a solicitous little mortuary man wearing platform shoes to boost his tininess. Streamed into a high pompadour, his hair glistened with hairspray, and he wore a fitted black suit with heavy gold chains lathered across his chest. He stood backlit in the doorway, like a Las Vegas apparition, the final theatrical wink that left my sister and I barely able to contain our laughter. In weeny script on a hospital napkin two afternoons before he died, my father had written, "Am I going yet?"

"Yes, daddy, you are," I'd said. No flinching there.

Then, two years later, after witnessing my mother as she was turned to powder behind the crematorium, and her gold fillings set aside, I took her packaged ashes to Pfieffer Beach, Big Sur, down the coast from where she'd grown up in San Francisco. My son stood watch on a giant boulder, as my daughter tossed her ashes onto me in grey handfuls. Naked, I dove under the waves to take her home—the closest we'd been outside her womb. If you say I was crazy, you'd be right. But here's the thing; I was also sane. She'd rarely been affectionate, and I remember an acute discomfort the few times she tried. So, on a cold day in May, I fixed her on me like a ghostly last word; we shivered in layers of grey on white. The bitter surf slammed my thighs, and then I dove into the sea, giving her back to the ocean she loved. I saved half of her for my sister.

So, I could have seen Bob lifeless in the mortuary basement. Two things stopped me. My daughter, Marah, reported a dream saying all that needed to be said, and 9/11 had happened twelve days before. I was working in a building nearby when the planes hit, so I was still staggering beneath images of the dead. My plan to fly across the country was out of the question. I found myself shaking in the middle of one sentence and crying in the next.

I wanted to watch the North Tower fall more than I can say. I can still hear the sound. Instinct saved me. I ran like hell. I hadn't known the escalating roar would send a huge cloud of ash and debris hurtling through the streets. I had no TV or computer images in my head. All news had come through the phone on my desk; muffled screams through my receiver had announced the South Tower's fall. As the wind raced up my back and my shoes flip flopped against my heels, I knew I had to put something tall and big between me and the raging crescendo. I collided with a fireman at the entrance of a building I've never been able to find since. We shouldered our way in. I don't remember his face, a smear with a helmet. How odd to consider his body was jammed against mine for one brief moment, so intimate and so anonymous, he and I forever out of reach outside this piece of history. His buddies came pouring in behind us. They stayed upstairs, waiting for orders in the large marble-floored foyer with its imposing concierge desk, as the vast room filled with black ash. I plunged into the basement where I met a Port Authority worker still wide-eyed from the implosion of his underground ticket kiosk, a casualty of the first plane's hit. No one was hurt down there, he said. We never knew each other's names. The names that mattered had already been ground to dust. They floated in the engulfing cloud, thickening the air. I poked my head upstairs. The firemen seemed alien in their gas masks as they flitted about like dark, misshapen moths. A woman with red hair and a mask with a long rubber snout shouted at me to stay below until it was safe. Like me, those firemen were the lucky ones.

The east face of the North Tower had looked so serene that glorious morning, smoke drifting up in lazy curls past the upper floors only blocks away from where I'd stood on Broadway, alone. I was advancing to meet my sister at Varick and Canal, which meant I was walking west, towards the World Trade Center, not away from it. My sister's voice had reported the second plane's hit, and ditto for the Pentagon. Rumors flew about the large room, leaping across cubicle walls. Cellphones were dead. I didn't ask for permission—I left. Hope for the North Tower's names had still been alive when I'd stepped off the elevator into the smoky lobby, and outside into the sky's overturned wastebasket, paper drifting down like fat snowflakes. Hands thrust water bottles and paper towels at me as I walked against the tide of mute people coming east, carrying briefcases and purses, heads and shoulders dusted white, until there was only the city and me.

A shoebox lid tucked under my arm that had been blown out of a Tower shop, landing intact and pristine in a doorway only blocks from a place that no longer existed. A cardboard print of a single open eye, a beautiful woman's eye that floated in a Magritte-like blue sky with puffy white clouds. *How surreal for a shoebox lid*, I thought. I can't say why I picked it up, but it seemed to mean something.

At Broadway, I felt too close. I'd already dropped down a block when I heard the deep rumble that chills my blood to this day. I knew what it meant. I turned to face the old world giving way to the new. I wanted to watch the tower fall in the same way I'd needed to carry my mother's ashes. *Be* there, together, in sympathy. The World Trade Center was a small city for all seasons with branching corridors; its ground floor had been a familiar home. I'd bought lipstick and eye shadow in Sephora, a pair of pants from The Gap the Christmas before, coffee, eaten food at the Chinese and Italian places, and upstairs, for over two years I'd done some significant personal therapy that had changed my life. The cavernous elevators had recessed plastic buttons that, when pressed, lifted smoothly skyward into large rooms where floor-to-ceiling windows did not open.

I recently heard about the shame some family members feel about those who jumped, as if there's a right way to die in a cataclysm. I want to put them on the window ledge with 1400° Fahrenheit at their backs and no exit, and see what they do. Let them choose to burn, as if there's any choice at all, or any difference.

Instead, the wind trilled up my spine with an enforcing speed, where it still hums. Can you imagine it? The groan magnified beyond all hearing on the inside, the mayhem of steel shattering concrete and glass, bodies colliding with desks and chairs, toilets ripped from the walls spiraling into the fiery murk of soap, towels, shoes, pens, rings, hands without limbs, teeth without mouths. Coffee cups, lunch bags, refrigerators, computers, the last calls home, the last everything ground to nothing in an incomprehensible roar. That night, on the Upper West Side, my sister and I rented the movie *Wit*. Emma Thompson's version of death from cancer seemed like the best antidote; a more reasonable, less violent death the size of one human being. I didn't know Bob would be next.

Bob died alone in the early hours, in Los Angeles. In Marah's dream, he died happy. He'd been reduced to the size of a little boy sitting in the middle of a huge hospital bed. His excess self had exploded, the unnecessary blood and fluids pooled around him on the floor, like a shallow swimming hole. He said, "I'm alright," and was smiling. Finally, after a lifetime of being more than he could handle, the levers behind the curtain were still. No more gaseous heads like the one in his favorite film, *The Wizard of Oz,* no more visits to hospital emergency rooms, where he used the visceral display of someone else's broken body to keep him from suicide. Bipolar, a self-medicating prescription drug abuser diagnosed too late, on and off lithium, he did find moments of equilibrium in his last few years, even as he drove himself into bankruptcy. The mind does what it does.

Bob's absence feels steadier than his presence ever did; the story no longer floats in its sea of synaptic possibilities. Synapse Technologies, Inc. was the name of his last business. Ten years before he died, we worked together in the bungalows behind the condemned, and now demolished, Ambassador Hotel where Bobby Kennedy was shot. I have a piece of the kitchen linoleum where Kennedy fell. Shortly before he lost his foothold in the visual effects world he'd helped to build, and began his slide, Bob had generously given me a job in L.A., mentoring me into a self-supporting life that led to a career in Internet design in New York.

I'm not a believer in the afterlife, or a God. I've learned the hard way that an authentic life doesn't come from someone else's notion of how to be. I strive to live well, inside nature's indifferent embrace. Let her galaxies spin and crash; I'm fine with the return to stardust. I prefer the bird that just flew into my bedroom as I'm writing. How will it find its way back through the narrow space it entered? The vast mystery of being is enough. The bird flies out. If we humans have a future, and it's looking doubtful, maybe science will find a version of me chugging along in a parallel universe one day. In ours, like death and love, suffering doesn't need a reason. It's with us like the sun rising, so why not make the best of it?

Did Bob believe in God? I don't know. We never talked about it. Neither one of us had been fully indoctrinated. I was nominally Episcopalian; he was Reform Jewish. We celebrated the holidays with his family, but that was more like feeding the blood connection. Those things feel real to me, history being carried forward in the flesh of my offspring. Mostly, we ate Nana's memorable brisket and kugel, and the men discussed sports while the children played. My place was in the kitchen.

During our marriage, I'd assumed God existed, but had never really put the question to myself. As a little girl, "give us this day, our daily bread" was my favorite phrase in the Lord's Prayer, because the feel of bread suffused my mouth, much in the same way the taste of spinach accompanied *The Little Engine That Could*. Very early on, I could see the fundamental hypocrisy, even as I sipped the poisonous subtexts and watched them play across the minister's dour face. I stayed out of its orthodox grip, but no girl child can escape religion's pervasive misogyny. I don't know what associations Bob had with his upbringing. I do know he believed in fear; he believed in his imagination, and he believed he would die like his father, which he did.

Consider this fading time frame: JFK's assassination marks our beginning, and 9/11, our end. Post-Thanksgiving 1963, shortly after the prancing horse behind the caisson and John-John holding Jacqueline's hand, with my family in disbelief and sullen in front of the TV, Bob called, asking for a date. He said we'd never met; I insisted we had. I was wrong. A stranger stood on the porch, clean cut, in khaki pants and a pullover sweater, button-down collar, blue cotton shirt. Later, he jokingly said he'd picked me out, bending over my locker in Dickson Art Center, asked around for my name and looked me up in the student files. I was a virgin about to lapse. I'd finally seen my mother's dictum to wait for the man I planned to marry for what it was—irrelevant. Bob drove a light blue VW and took me for sushi on Sawtelle Ave. in West L.A., where I learned to use chopsticks. He introduced me to Seymour, who showed us slides of the Watts Towers.

Bob opened me to a vital world of art and jazz. Bebop was a word I hadn't known. Coltrane, Miles, and Coleman were playing live in the L.A. clubs. The Beatles, Little Richard, Chuck Berry, and The Temptations usurped the radio waves. Dylan and Joan Baez. The Grateful Dead. Dancing in a loft near the beach. In Westwood, at the Ferus Gallery: Warhol's Campbell Soup cans on white pedestals, Rauschenberg's washed looking, bloody collages, Jasper John's flags and paintbrushes. Bob filmed a Claes Oldenburg happening in the Pan Pacific Auditorium parking lot; car headlights trained on chunks of ice strewn across the asphalt, and fat fabric popsicles. I wore a pair of super-tight olive green corduroy pants with leather thongs laced partway up the sides, skin showing through, a burgundy velvet top, and a necklace of dyed seeds. In San Francisco, we visited friends and hung out with Ray Anderson, who ran the light shows at Fillmore West, his house crammed with memorabilia. I couldn't sleep from the theatrical visions staging themselves in my brain, light shows of my own, and no way out into the world that I could see, unable to share them with Bob or with anyone. Country Joe and the Fish, Big Brother and the Holding Company, no Janis (there was only one), but Cream loud in the hall. Grass, LSD, mescaline, but never with Bob, not once—he preferred cocaine. Later, Janis at the Shrine Auditorium in L.A., getting down under swags of necklaces, a grand and furious voice, its clock ticking, the motel room waiting. Bob lived in Beverly Glen Canyon with his roommate, Pat O'Neill, an avant-garde filmmaker. Bob and I had met as they were finishing their final edit of a Kodalith film on Venice Beach called, *By the Sea*. Their digs were filthy. I cleaned the place top to bottom. Thus did I start to lay down the tracks of the woman qualified to take Bob's mother's place. Bob made messes; his mother cleaned them up. She did this until the day she died. What did I know? I was not yet a person. I was a ball of heat and possibility, with absolutely nowhere to go, terrified of living my dreams while blacks marched from Selma to Montgomery.

What is a person, anyway? It seems to me I'm a ragtag collection of memories, a happening of randomly recalled events and momentary actions whose wholeness can't be known, more like the persistent idea of an evanescent process. Ditto for a marriage. From a distance, you might see a landscape if I can conjure one, but up close, Bob and I dissolve into daubs of paint. So, yes, I'm down the hole, all right, tearing alongside the white rabbit, but off to see what? An information flux clogged with fragmentary pieces. If there's a Queen, I'd sure like to meet her. Really.

Bob seemed like a person. He proposed to me in my parent's house in Brentwood, Los Angeles, in a guest bedroom. I remember the room in shadows. Carmelina Ave. north of

Sunset Blvd. I have no idea why he chose that moment. Something in the house he saw, or the way I looked? It didn't feel planned. No ring, just the sudden question, him pushing me onto the bed in what had been my sister's room. I knew nothing about myself at 20, so I said yes. *No* was not a word I knew how to use. *No* would lead where? To terrifying unknown places, like making decisions on my own, and a life directed by me, to what end? How, when my future, like my body, wasn't mine? Bob knew where *yes* would lead. "Fear is my best motivator," he said. It remained a true statement.

I lost my virginity in front of the fireplace in the rented Beverly Glen Canyon house. I'd worried it would hurt, but it didn't. No hymen, after all. Probably broken while riding my horse. Or did the man who twice molested me when I was 8 take care of it? Don't remember any pain, only humiliation and fear, and the probing finger. Bob was sweet and tender. But then the lovemaking went in other directions. It was full of weird surprises that included whips. I had a faux attitude of acceptance about everything. Anything goes in the bedroom, I convinced myself, dismissing my own tastes. I was afraid to have any. No wonder I couldn't orgasm, until finally, a year into our marriage, I confessed that he scared me. He'd whispered on more than one occasion he wanted to burn my labia with cigarettes. Had I ever asked myself what I was feeling when I'd pretended to hang from a ceiling that couldn't take my weight as he halfheartedly hit me with a belt, not really hurting me, but wanting to fantasize that he was? No, I'd repressed all that. I was taught to repress things early on. You might not feel loved, you might be abused, but what the hell do you do with that stuff when you're a child, except find ways to make it normal?

If whipping was exciting to Bob, it wasn't exciting to me. I thought it was ridiculous. What possible connection to eroticism and passion could it have? I rode horses and read books, so whether I had a self or not, I needed a man as compelling as horseflesh on the move. I knew how to use a whip, but a dick brain swinging a whip, like in some squirrely porno flick, had zero erotic allure. But then again, I'm not a man. What the dick was attached to was the only point I cared about. I had my bookish upper-middle class requirements: tall, dark, broad shouldered, an athletic man at ease with his body, strong and virile, intellectually alive, gifted, with heart, integrity, vulnerability, courage, wit, talent, common sense, and a future. Money didn't count; it would come. I had no itemized list of my own qualities, of course. Only my charms mattered, the accommodating shape of a woman built to hold her man's fantasies. Rhett Butler was my model, but Bob was no Rhett Butler. I was no Scarlett O'Hara either. What was up with me? My mother had used the strap often enough. I'd almost let it turn me into a liar, until at 10 years old, I decided to take the punishment. Now I see I became a liar, anyway. I may have stopped the small lies; it was the big ones I missed. Was it the Victorian abuse, along with the million other weird bits curled up inside our family's DNA that anchored me to the ceiling, mute and yielding? I never did become a fan. No judgment about others here, and hopefully none about me. My sexual nature is pure animal, horse and stable, the smell of manure, sweat, and leather. A bed is not necessary, and please don't tie me to it or truss me up like a chicken. But I craved the illusion of love.

Love was the one thing I never felt from my parents, although I do have an unabashed lust for the penis if it's the right one. As a 3-year-old, I'd crawl under my parents' bedcovers just to see it and, yes, be excited. The one time I got Bob out of the car onto the ground in Big Sur, he looked like an alien lost among the bushes, dressed in white. His lovemaking was about imagination and fantasy. He made drawings that would get him off, seeking release from whatever haunted him. I wanted to feel the monkey. No wonder our sex life never made it into the trees. We both needed someone else.

When Bob was a boy, his father, Sonny, took him out of town to watch the trains. Bob was nuts about them, and memorialized his experience in a little gem of an animation film called, *Freight Yard Symphony,* his first. They walked to some remote place where Sonny left Bob close to the tracks and returned to the top of the embankment. The train hurtled by, and Bob found himself on his stomach, scrabbling for bits of grass, desperate to keep from being pulled beneath the wheels. He told me how frightened he was at the sucking roar, how he fought for his life, and how his father looked down at him, laughing, oblivious. Laughing like my father had laughed at me? Did Sonny know he was putting his son in danger? It seems to be a question that remains unanswered. The family left Milwaukee for Los Angeles after their apartment burned down. When Sonny wasn't golfing on the weekends, he was having a hard time making a living. He had two heart attacks in the hospital, and died bankrupt. The day before he died, he and Bob had their first intimate man-to-man talk. Sonny cried, admitting that he was a failure. Bob went to see him the next day, but Sonny was gone. Bob said to me, "The book that best describes me is *What Makes Sammy Run.*" I've still not read it; I don't need to.

We gave a couple of big dinner parties at the Beverly Glen house before we were married. Leonard Nimoy, my acting coach (pre-*Star Trek*), came with his then-wife, Sandy, as did our circle of acting friends. Years later, he married Susan Bay, with whom I'd written a little play when we were 18. I cooked my mother's beef stroganoff and cleaned the house again. Wasn't this my job, the one I'd been brought up to do, despite my mother's admonishments to acquire a skill that would give me a living? What did I know from earning a living? Did she earn one? I'd babysat and worked behind the counter at the Brentwood Pharmacy, and in the art department store at UCLA, enough to buy a slick black Chevy convertible, but what did that prove? The only living being made was by my father, John Dehner, an actor, and he didn't care much about what happened to me. He acknowledged my Thespian talents, but he didn't want me messing around in his world. I doubted myself too much to forge ahead. Once, when I was still thinking acting might be something I could do, he came to a performance, and when I wept on cue, I heard him suck in his breath and turn in his seat. "How did you do that?" he asked, afterwards, incredulous.

Marry? Hell yes, I was off his hands. He was out front, watering, standing in the driveway and holding the hose when I told him Bob and I were engaged, and had already had sex. I think my mother had instructed me to tell him. "Now you won't be able to wear white at your wedding," he said. No congratulations that I remember, just the water plopping on the driveway's asphalt apron ringed with ferns. Years later, after divorcing my mother and marrying her former friend, he said to me, before a party they were about to give, "You can decorate the place," as in, "Be all that you are to me. Be the ornament in the room." Chalk it up to being a daughter, instead of the son he wanted. Chalk it up to him having been abused by his father. Chalk it up to what he didn't think of when he thought about women. It all helped to generate the confusion I felt for the longest time. When Bob was talking to me about the presence of an absence, he was talking about me.

The photos Bob took of me at The Seven Gables Inn, the night before we got married, show a somber woman. Something is wrong. After the Watts riots in 1965 killed our plans for a wedding at the earthquake-proof Towers, we went up the coast to Pacific Grove to be married by a Justice of the Peace, in a snug house behind a white picket fence ringed with daisies. Our witnesses were his wife, a German shepherd, and a neighbor in curlers. The wife's makeup ended at her jawline; she wore pedal pushers and Springolator shoes with glued-on plastic flowers. The neighbor bawled on the couch. A marriage at 21 was a way to feel safe in the short term and avoid the trials of being alone. Bob would carry me into the future. How could I know that being carried would only confirm how helpless I was, and foster an anger only dependency can create?

Now I can see clearly the fantasy that was meant to repair my childhood, but at the time, it hadn't even registered in the haze of my consciousness. The images were present, but, like everything else, they stayed wrapped inside vague feelings I couldn't articulate. I wanted to be happy. I wanted something that I didn't have inside me. A sweet home with at least three children running in and out, a garden dizzy with peonies, hip friends, and a hip life—as in cool, educated, up with the latest in art and literature, travel, great food, and conversation, delicious sex, and a loving husband who adored his children, and who adored me. I wasn't supposed to create this life, mind you, since I didn't believe I had the power to create anything except a dinner. These fantasized bits and pieces were to be given to me like magical gifts—by Bob, I suppose. How unfair. I was a child cocooned inside an impossible wish. I was being everything I knew how to be.

Bob began editing *Seven Second Love Affair,* a drag-racing documentary he'd shot with Rick "The Iceman" Stewart, one of drag racing's pioneers. We'd hung out with Rick and Linda in their garage, and gone with them to the track where smoke poured off the wheels, the starting lights counting down, red to green. Life happened. Marriage happened. The photographer, Jerome Liebling, brought us to Minneapolis so Bob could teach at the University of Minnesota. It was my first trip east. Although my father had grown up in Hastings-on-Hudson, New York, he'd never taken us to visit. Both of my parents were mysteriously dismissive of the East Coast. At one point, while still in high school, I planned a trip to Europe. I would go all by myself and rent a motorbike. Brochures for freighters and maps were scattered in piles on our living room floor, where I sat cross-legged. I couldn't imagine making it happen, not really. I needed someone else to propel me through all the doubts and fears, and show me how to book the tickets. Our family travel had taken us to the Southwest and Indian country, where a Zuni child is named after me, and then several times to a ranch in the High Sierras not far from the ghost town, Bodie, north of Bishop. Riding alone in the mountains, across pastures in the rain, with rainbow trout dangling from the pommel was my idea of bliss. Here is where I could feel myself in the wild animal that prowled my dreams. On insomniac nights, when wanting to run away was so intense I could barely stay in bed, I knew where to run: up to the little cabin hidden in the pines high above Twin Lakes where no one would find me. I'd fish for trout; I'd have an adventure. Instead, I fell asleep.

The Victorian houses of Minneapolis were new to me—the old smell of them, the creaky wooden floors, curved banisters, and elm leaves turning yellow against the black branches in the October rain. Jerry and his wife, Phyllis, welcomed us, fed and entertained us, and helped us find an apartment on Humboldt Ave. South. Bad things were happening to me. I felt unmoored and had no sense of what to do or who to be. The world was too big. I was afraid to audition for the Guthrie Theater. Flash, the kitten we'd adopted, who rode in our Volvo curled up in the hood of Bob's winter jacket behind his head, died of feline leukemia. From the back porch—the porch was a novel experience for a Southern California girl—I watched Bob dig a small grave in the frozen earth with a pick he'd either bought or borrowed. Snow for a whole season, Salvation Army Store purchases that included a Wurlitzer jukebox, a stack of 78s, a carved oak barber chair, and the smell of wet leaves. Then Bob left, walking away from his second-semester commitment. He could do that, no problem. He went back to L.A. to finish the drag-racing film, leaving Jerry high and dry, and me in Minneapolis, where I was alone for the first time in my life. A good thing, as it turned out. I was cast in a Durrenmatt play at Theater St. Paul, my first professional role. That summer, a man jumped out of the bushes, exposing himself, as I walked around the Lake of the Isles. This time, I chased the fucker all the way back to his car, his fat ass humping it down the sidewalk. I was tired of men exposing themselves to me on beaches and sidewalks, as if I were a siren calling out to the damaged corners of their minds. Still not seeing mine.

Before we were married, Bob put together an exhibit at UCLA built around people's cherished artifacts. I was there when a teacher reluctantly handed over a letter written in pencil by a special needs student most dear to her. I'd watched her nervously resist his request. I'd listened to him persuade her, soothing her fears until she gave in. At the exhibit's opening, an enlarged photo of the letter hung on the wall; both the boy's name and hers had been erased. She freaked. I felt sick. I thought, why didn't you simply cover the names before taking the picture, Bob? Why destroy something so precious that doesn't belong to you? But Bob had no idea what he'd done. To him, the image was everything, the only thing, not the person to whom it had meaning.

And there it was, a piercing moment like others before it, and so many after, asking me to honor my forbidden thoughts: what am I doing, why am I with a man who does this to a woman, or to anyone? Just like the other times, I couldn't pursue the answer. What right did I have to my doubts, and what would I do with them? I'd already said I would marry; it was a done deal. Besides, nothing that had happened to me had ever been undone, so what choice was there? I didn't consider what *not* answering the question said about my character, and what the consequences might be.

This is the Kirsten mute before her parents when she was 8, feeling the heat of the older man next to her, knowing what he will do, and Bob, at once both a generous mentor and user of people, running for his life, straight towards the target he's made of his father's death. Many times, these threads played themselves out in our life together. Bob on cocaine, popping pills, and building a fine career; me getting sick and building a house we never lived in, tennis courts down the road, a Mercedes in the driveway, two children struggling to keep up with their parents' delusions, divorce inevitable.

I'll tell you who I've been. Most of my life, I've been the child afraid to tell my parents who are about to go off for a late afternoon horseback ride in Griffith Park that the man standing next to me is going to do something to me again. I don't know what he'll do or where he'll do it, exactly. As it turns out, on the other side of the trail, in the grassy park where men in whites are playing cricket, underneath a large tree with exposed roots and a thick trunk to provide cover. John Sherman is an actor, like my father, an Australian, probably dead now. One can only hope. They'd met making the movie, *Plymouth Adventure*. He'd paid attention to me at one or more of my parents' parties. I wasn't used to this; I adored him for it. I remember one party, sitting on his lap, thrilled, thinking he loved me. No one loved me. Pedophiles know who to target; he'd probably been abused himself. The first time he'd molested my sister and me, we'd waited for him by the living room window to see his car pull into our driveway in Encino, orange blossoms off the trees below. He'd arrived late. We'd never gone away like this, without our parents, and were over the moon with excitement. He drove us to Hollywood to see a movie, and then to his apartment for lunch, where he did us both on the couch, me on one side of him, my sister on the other, one hand on a children's book, his other elsewhere. Shifting hands, one in, one out, he read to us, leaving our scent on the pages.

It could have begun at the movie in the flickering dark, where I think he forced the dread that has been with me for a lifetime. Or had that gnarly bloom been planted when I was sent to a foster home at two when my sister was about to be born, where I threw up in a strange woman's lap and the hollow dreams began with long tin roofs leaking rain? Who knows? How reliable are these memories? It doesn't matter; these are the ones. A vague recollection of the light from an open refrigerator door, sharp words out of nowhere insinuating danger, and me, polite and false to the core, holding on to the round table with our plates of sandwiches, adrift in the viscous fluid of my imagination, the only refuge between me and whatever end there might be. Caught between wanting to get away, and hiding my fear, I complied. What else? It's what girls do, and boys too. Neither of us told our parents. These may have been the man's instructions, and these, it turns out, are the instructions I've lived by.

This time, I know what the man wants. It's after school, and my parents mean it as a good surprise. I'm afraid to disappoint. I stand on the trail with his dark body to my left, both of us looking up at them sitting their horses like a pair of smiling cutouts. We're creepy, Mr. Sherman and I. We both know I feel powerless to prevent what's going to happen and will not tell. My father leans over his pommel, smiling at me. I stare back soundlessly. I will him to not go, for something to break that isn't me. I want him to see the impossible, that this one time I'm right, and he and mommy are wrong. This man is not my friend.

Words fill my mouth like a thousand scrabbling animals. Who am I to let them out into the plain air? Smiles will drop like stones and there will be hell to pay. Mr. Sherman will deny it, act shocked, say I'm lying. What if they believe him? What then? It's a scene I don't want to imagine. I've been blamed before for things I didn't do. I know where the belt hangs in the closet.

Speak, speak not, speak dart like bats inside a cave.

My father straightens up and swings his horse around. My mother follows and they head down the trail, backs swaying in the indifferent late afternoon light. The bats die. My faith in words dies. I will follow Mr. Sherman, whose hand is already sliding up my arm. Silence becomes the lie I will repeat in countless circumstances, despite my promise not to. And here thrums a dim and tautly woven thread deep in the tapestry: the struggle to find my voice, to trust myself, to speak the truth.

My sister is the one who finally tells. I'd said how he'd gone into my pants, how I'd lain stiff on my stomach, while he'd wormed his way around with his coarse, blunt fingers. I don't remember talking to my parents, or being comforted, just the trip to the Beverly Hills police station where, wearing my lucky navy blue cardigan and jeans, I gave a report that we never spoke of again. My parents' instructions, 1952.

With Bob, it began so sweetly in the blue VW. It was our second date and we were parked on the wide apron off my parents' driveway, the taste of sushi and soy sauce lingering. We sat there, silent, with the motor off, and I knew he wanted to kiss me and was uncertain, so I reached across and ran the tips of my fingers down his cheek. I made it easy; he made his move. I liked him; there was something. Then, I couldn't stop, as if having my first lover inevitably meant marriage, which it didn't, not really, since ours wasn't my longed-for sultry dance in *Picnic,* because he carried a doubt about himself I could feel and taste, and yet he loved me, or something like that. Or, maybe just because Sammy was on the run and I was part of the picture in his head; the girl at the top of the list he'd made of the girls he'd wanted to date, thinking I was beyond his reach, he said, and I wasn't. I was in a place of change, and here was the man it had to be about, since change couldn't be about me. That was my failure. Bob wanted me as half of a working team. He kept offering me a place at his side, but I couldn't show up, not in the way he envisioned, because

I was sure I'd die if I did, since it didn't take long to feel like a rat inside his cage. Now that I know the cage was also built by me, I wonder what would have happened if I *had* shown up. I might have found myself there, or left sooner. Maybe not.

He was who he was too. One meal, 1969, I was still trying to plump up my hazy adolescent fantasy of a retro-perfect Fifties wife. Julia Child's insouciance, the roasted pig flying off the counter to the floor as she said, "Oops," picked it up, and went right on in front of the cameras offered a path through domestic service and isolation that included humor and sensory delight. He'd brought his secretary as a surprise. I was pregnant with our first child, Joshua, pleased to have a moment with Bob, who rarely came home, even if I had to share it. I'd made a *coq au vin*, a trim little shape I carved into pieces and served onto a plate next to the green beans with sliced almonds. We sat at his grandmother's wooden table. As I happily ladled the sauce and passed the plates, chatting away, I didn't know they'd just fucked in the little green Porsche he wouldn't let me drive. I didn't learn of this betrayal until well after we were divorced, one betrayal among many, as it turned out. He wasn't there day after day, year after year, until my anger grew in such proportion, there was only rage leading to my own affair eight years later, which in turn led to divorcing Bob, marrying again, and moving to New York with my children. Then there was nothing, or so it seemed for a long time.

On 9/11, I left the shoebox lid in a public phone booth, where I was trying to reach my sister. I'd arrived at the park where we'd agreed to meet and saw the familiar benches, but my mind couldn't place it. Holding out a laminated downtown map, I kept asking passersby to show me where I was. Then I saw Sheila striding towards me in her bright green jacket, and

I bolted into the crosswalk to meet her, leaving the shoebox lid behind. Its loss has haunted me ever since.

At first, I thought it was precious because it was the only tangible evidence I had from 9/11. It was so much more. I'd been carrying the image of a woman's eye surviving disaster, a fragile paper icon of female perception. She was *my* eye, the voice of *my* perceptions. She was woman seeing what too many men don't see: the impact of their ungoverned appetites. The results are war, terrorism, Sharia Law, capitalized greed—wherever tender impulses are brutalized in favor of aggression. How many virgins were the 9/11 terrorists promised as reward for their jihad? My *Moorish Illusionary Fantasy* poster has acquired new meanings. The Arab dancer has been made the cause of jealous argument, even though she herself is nothing, only a coin for barter in the fight over male supremacy, an ancient vessel for the blame men lay on women, because they can't, or won't, control themselves. A symbol, too, of women who collude, who agree we have less worth, dancing their dance out of fear and ignorance, playing their female parts for gain, and the illusion of protection. There is no protection. We are in it together. Men pursue their territorial imperatives while women sew up the psyches of their children or bury their cherished bodies. And men call women weak? I'd brought out from the debris of man-made catastrophe the unsullied image of a woman's eye floating free, one of peace, beauty, and unflinching love calling me to myself—only to abandon her, once again, as so many women do.

9/11 marks the end of Bob and me. When he was finally removed from the cardiac intensive unit and I could reach him, I called and asked the nurse to put the phone to his ear, and tell him to blink in response. I'd been told he couldn't talk. He blinked, she said. I explained 9/11 had kept me from coming earlier, that I loved him and soon would be in L.A. to see him. Blink. Blink. The last conversation, until now. Maybe the nurse was humoring me, because my son says he was non-communicative before he ever left intensive care. No one knew what happened to him and why he suddenly went blank. Still, they say hearing is the last to go. I sang to my father the last night he was alive, and if I'd been there, I'd have sung to Bob.

The thing about a marriage is it never ends, even with divorce. It's always in you. I've discovered this while writing these pages. Who could have known thinking about Bob's death would have led me down this path where the knotted threads could suddenly loosen and patterns emerge, the mirage of self coalescing into understanding?

On Christmas, 1996, Bob mailed me a tape. He called it "Precious Images," and tucked inside the box sleeve were these words:

> *Kirsten,*
>
> *I once thought that creating images was a substitute for creating and nurturing relationships, and held that fallacy so close, that I couldn't see...Well, I've grown up...When you watch this, remember that someone far away still holds you very "precious."*
> *Love,*
> *Bob*

The rabbit has turned the corner and vanished, coattails flickering past the hedge, leaving me alone in the garden where I belong. For you see, there's no blame; this is not a victim's story. Bob loved me. I know this. On the eve of our separation in 1979, he played Joe Cocker's *You Are So Beautiful* over and over again. He didn't want to go; didn't want us to end. What I don't know is if I ever allowed myself to truly love him. Since most of what happens between people can't be known in any way that can be measured, why not make something new from something old? Bob is here, as close to me as he can ever be or ever was. No breath is necessary other than mine. As a man who loved his images, he will like this: rabbits out of hats, sleights of hand. Magic was his province, top hat, glove, and cane sashaying across your eyeballs; these were his studio's icons.

I will take his hand in mine, right here on this page. You can share this with us, for you are here too, as much as anyone can be anywhere. Bob and I are in a place we once were, where he took me out to dinner one evening when I was 19. I was dressed up and so was he. He knew how to dress. I'd stood next to him in his favorite men's store, maybe a week before, or was it a week after, or a month, a day in some year before we were married, as he picked out a new tie. I knew nothing about ties, and had never thought about them before. He'd held several against different shirts. So this is how you pick a tie, I'd thought, a small wake-up connecting me to the world of men in the dry shine of patterned silk, a touch of peacock. The band starts to play. He looks at me in that way he had, a concentration of sweetness and desire that only scared me then, because where would it lead? I had no means to protect myself, or so I thought. We set down our wine glasses. He takes me in his arms, and we swing around the floor, cheek-to-cheek, still-tender bodies pressed up against each other, our children not yet imagined. It's not the dance in *Picnic,* and it doesn't need to be. I don't shrink before his gaze; the smell of him doesn't call on unknown fears, for everything I can and cannot know of Bob is already here, in me. Fearful flesh of the child who felt untouched by love is no longer an impediment to feeling. Bob left himself a long time ago, but he didn't leave me. I take him in my arms, now fully present, and we dance.

Dear Bob, We dance.

CHAPTER 9

THE BRUTAL MURDER OF MR. HYDE

~ ANNETTE BIRCHARD[1] ~

[Editors' note: This chapter is unique in this volume in that it was written a mere two months after the death of the author's ex. Thus she writes without the benefit of hindsight and years of reflection that the other chapter authors have experienced. We include this chapter gratefully, perceiving that Annette's words open an important window onto the tornado of fresh, raw, immediate grief and the raging winds of emotions it draws into its vortex. The author does not try to sugarcoat; rather she grits her teeth and chooses to be honest with her readers and herself in both her better, and her pettier moments. If you are presently whirling around in that tornado as you read, perhaps this chapter will serve you best of all right now, while later you may find that other, more reflective chapters will match or inform you more deeply as your process unfolds.]

My ex-husband, Jeff, was brutally murdered in June of 2012. On the morning of Jeff's death, my daughter, Nicole, called me at work and told me that Jeff's daughter, Laura, had called to tell her that the house Jeff was living in with his girlfriend, Mary, had been broken into, and that both Jeff and Mary had been bludgeoned with a crowbar. Before I could respond, Nicole got another call on her cellphone and said it was Laura. Nicole said she would call me back. Just 2 minutes later, Nicole called again and she was sobbing. She said, "He's dead, Mom—Jeff's dead, he's dead." My initial reaction was deep sympathy

---

1   Names changed in this chapter.

and heartache for Nicole; as her mom, I wanted so much to be able to shield her from the pain. For myself, I felt stunned and completely emotionless. All I could think to say was, "Nicole, I'm so sorry for you, my heart aches for you. I wish I knew the perfect thing to say." Nicole left work soon after she talked to me, and drove to the town where Jeff had lived. Jeff's twin daughters, Lindsey and Laura, were there, and Nicole stayed with them at Jeff's brother's house for a few days.

For the first two days after Jeff's death, I stayed emotionless. His death was constantly on my mind, but I just didn't feel anything inside. I really wanted to cry, but the tears didn't come. On the third day, anger smacked my heart hard. Memories of our marriage came from nowhere, directly to the forefront of my mind. I wasn't grieving a loss; I was pissed at Jeff and what our relationship could have been.

Nicole called me every evening and relayed information about the circumstances surrounding Jeff's death as the police talked to his family. Jeff had been living with Mary in her house. Mary's 20-year-old daughter was living there too. Jeff was asleep on the couch, Mary was in her and Jeff's bedroom, and Mary's daughter was in another bedroom. The daughter's ex-boyfriend broke into the house around 3 a.m. and bludgeoned both Jeff and Mary with a crowbar while they were sleeping. The daughter was unharmed. Jeff died soon after being transported to the hospital. Mary survived her injuries and is in a rehabilitation facility—her ability to recover from her traumatic brain injuries will be unknown for quite some time. We have no information on a possible motive.

Jeff's murder was high-profile in the small town where he lived, and so was covered extensively by the local newspaper and television stations. I read all of the online newspaper articles about his murder, along with the comments that people made on the articles. One person described Jeff as kind and gentle. Another person said he was, "nice, easy-going, funny, and the best neighbor." Yet another talked about how "genuine and sincere" Jeff was, saying that he was always accepting of everyone exactly as they were. I was FURIOUS when I read those comments about Jeff because they certainly didn't describe the same man I was remembering.

Coping: A few days after Jeff's murder, I called my long-time friend, Carrie, to express my absolute rage about the newspaper article comments I was reading. Carrie is really the only person who knows exactly how badly Jeff treated me through the years I was with him. She has proved to be a wonderful sounding board, helping me to channel my rage into more productive ways of thinking. Other people didn't know the same Jeff that I knew, and what other people are saying about him *does not change the way he treated me.* Most people who knew Jeff found him charming, funny, caring, and genuine. They would have needed extensive involvement with him over time to discover how much of a jerk he actually was. When I left Jeff, I made the right decision for Nicole and me. It will take some time for me to forgive Jeff for a lot of things, but Carrie suggested that maybe *because he's dead,* it will be easier for me find the closure that I need. There is definitely no way that Jeff can hurt me again.

Jeff's memorial service was on a Monday. Nicole and I spent the Saturday and Sunday before the service talking about Jeff and what we remembered about him. My tears started to flow as I listened to Nicole talk about her memories, and tell me that she felt as if a huge part of her had been ripped away. Nicole viewed Jeff as an important part of her life, so the heartache I continue to feel for her is unbearable. She is deeply distressed that Jeff will not be part of her future.

I did attend Jeff's memorial service, yet hesitated at first because I had so much anger in my heart, and I wasn't sure that I was ready to "pay my respects" to someone who had treated me so badly. Nicole wanted me to attend—she felt strongly that Jeff would have wanted me to be there. I decided to attend because Nicole helped me to realize that Jeff's memorial service would not happen when it was convenient for me, and I wouldn't have the option in the future to attend it after I sorted through all the emotions that had yet to hit me.

Another reason I hesitated to attend Jeff's service was because I wasn't sure what role I played as Jeff's ex-wife, given that he had been living with Mary. I knew that Mary would be part of Jeff's service because they had been brutally attacked at the same time. I questioned myself as to whether or not I was ready to see Jeff and Mary together in pictures at the service, and I wasn't sure what my feelings would be when I saw members of Mary's family there. But one of Jeff's brothers called and asked me to attend the service. That call solidified my decision to go.

At the service, all of Jeff's family greeted me as if I was still a member of their family. I was grateful that I had the opportunity to express my sympathy and shock at Jeff's sudden demise. At the service, Jeff's sister-in-law hugged me right away, and when I told her how sorry I was, her eyes welled up with tears, and she said, "You loved him too." One of Jeff's brothers hugged me for a long time and he really, really cried. Very few words were exchanged between us—when I looked into his eyes, I could see that he just couldn't find any words to express what he was feeling. Another of Jeff's brothers put his arm around me and together, we watched a slideshow of pictures that Jeff's daughters had created. Some pictures were of Jeff and Mary together; viewing them with Jeff's brother's arm around me made seeing them easier than I had thought it would be. One of Jeff's nephews, whom I had been particularly close to, hugged me long and hard. It had always been somewhat of a joke that this nephew looked exactly like Jeff. I reminded him again of the similarity—that was almost unbearable for him to hear and the tears rolled down his face. I'm hanging on to all those moments at Jeff's service because they have helped me cope with one of the main issues that I'm struggling with now: the fact that Jeff had a relationship with Mary at the time of his death. Jeff's family made me feel as though my role in Jeff's life has not been forgotten, and that I am still a member of their family.

Jeff and I were high school sweethearts—we kept in touch for a few years after we graduated. Eventually, we lost track of one another and connected again when I came to town for our 20-year high school reunion. Jeff was divorced and had twin daughters, aged 10 (25 years old now). I was divorced and had one daughter, aged 6 (21 years old now). We never had children together. We were married for ten years and separated for a year before our divorce was final in 2007. During our separation, we lived 150 miles away from each other in separate states. Yet we kept in touch, and for the first three years after our divorce, Jeff and I visited each other off and on. After Nicole graduated from high school in 2009, she went to a community college in the town where our blended family had lived. During her first year of college, Nicole lived with Jeff and Laura in the house that we had shared. Jeff stopped communicating with me some time in 2010, when he started a relationship with Mary. We both knew Mary from high school.

When I went back for my 20-year high school reunion in Sioux City, Iowa, I was living in Denver. I had been divorced from Nicole's dad for five years and I had been thinking about moving to a smaller town. Nicole's dad was never too interested in seeing her on a regular basis, and I longed for a shorter commute to work, a closer daycare, less-crowded grocery stores, movie theaters, and parks; and kid-friendly festivals. I hadn't thought of moving back to Iowa—I was only feeling a need to relocate to a less-populated area. After connecting with Jeff while in town for the reunion, the love sparks were flying high between us. We talked on the phone every day after the reunion, and I started to think that Sioux City would be a good place for Nicole and me to live.

Six months after the reunion, I secured a job in Sioux City and moved back. The size of the town was perfect, and the daily grind of getting here and there for work and entertainment disappeared. Jeff and I rented a small house with only two bedrooms and one bathroom. It was a challenge with five people, but Jeff's and my relationship started strong, and we soon both felt that we were ready to take the plunge into marriage and make a lifelong commitment to each other and our children. I felt that my decision to marry again would benefit Nicole immediately—Lindsey, Laura, and Nicole considered each other as sisters right from the get-go. Their devotion to each other has never wavered. In addition, Jeff's immediate family all lived in Sioux City. They welcomed us with open arms, and treated Nicole as if she were a biological member of their family. I felt very lucky to have found a family whose members would share themselves so completely with Nicole and me.

I know I will be trying to sort out many of my feelings for quite some time. An important part of my history, all the way back to high school, has been taken away from me. I'm angry because I'm still wishing for a relationship with Jeff as *it should have been*. Moments of grief, tears, and heartache for myself have yet to surface. I can't cry when I think of my relationship with Jeff. I can only cry when I realize how much Jeff's death has hurt Nicole, and when I think about how much grief Jeff's family expressed at his memorial service. I'm still remembering how mean Jeff could be sometimes—the best description I can come up with to describe Jeff is "Dr. Jekyll and Mr. Hyde." Within Jeff, there existed two distinct person-alities, and I'm still struggling with the Mr. Hyde side.

The Mr. Hyde side of Jeff was oppressive. Soon after we were married, it became clear that Jeff had some serious personal issues that were a constant thorn in the side of our marriage. He was a very angry person deep inside; he struggled with anger on a daily basis. Jeff suffered from severe hearing loss that caused him to be paranoid about what was being said about him in the conversations he could not hear. He was an alcoholic who never saw that his personality changed from Dr. Jekyll to Mr. Hyde when he drank. Most significantly for me, Jeff never took control over his ex-wife's ability to manipulate him—he allowed her to dictate what his life was like with their daughters.

The Dr. Jekyll side of Jeff was amazing! I always knew that deep down inside his soul, there was a kind, gentle, and compassionate man. That's why I stayed with him so long, continuously trying to work on our marriage. Sometimes we'd talk for hours about our spiritual purpose on earth and what we thought it was like "on the other side" after death. We remembered times in high school together, and shared funny stories about ourselves when we were growing up. We talked about everything imaginable. He was my husband, lover, soulmate, cheerleader, and best friend.

When Jeff and I got married, I knew that my yearly salary was thousands of dollars more than his salary, and that he was living paycheck to paycheck, and didn't have extra material things. I trusted that he would be able to pay his child support, and provide for Lindsey and Laura when their expenses were not covered by his support. Before we married, I asked Jeff about his credit card debt. I didn't ask to see billing statements. He told me he didn't owe money to anyone, and I believed him. After our marriage, we combined our money into one bank account. When the rental house lease was up, we purchased a house that provided each of our daughters with individual bedrooms. We applied for a mortgage loan together. It was only when the loan officer ran a credit report on Jeff that I learned of his terrible credit rating, the enormous amount due on his credit cards, and an outstanding fine to the city for a Driving Under the Influence (DUI) charge he had pled guilty to 3 years before. Obviously, his name could not be on the mortgage.

I knew that the 10% down payment on the house would come from my mutual fund, but I was still disappointed that the mortgage was in my name only because it felt as though we didn't really share the house. I also knew that the expense of beds, sheets, blankets, and storage shelves for his daughters would come from my savings because before the rental house, Jeff had been living in a one-bedroom apartment with only a sofa-sleeper for Lindsey and Laura. They didn't have a place to store any personal items. After we closed on the house, I immediately paid off Jeff's credit cards and the DUI fine. Now that I was married to Jeff, I didn't want to take a chance that his bills would affect my excellent credit rating. I also paid afterschool care expenses for Laura and Lindsey when the provider informed me that Jeff had not paid these expenses for the past several months. When we jointly filed our taxes the first year, I found out that Jeff had not filed taxes for the past several years. I was able to file as a "non-injured spouse." Half of our refund went to pay his past taxes; the other half went into our joint bank account for the next five years.

Jeff drove a jalopy that broke down after our first year of marriage and was too expensive to repair. He found a used truck that he wanted, so I took money from my mutual fund and gave him a cashier's check to cover the cost of the truck. He didn't have my name put on the title. After a year, the truck's transmission went kaput and he needed another vehicle. I didn't see any other option except to finance another used vehicle because at the bare minimum, he needed a means to get to work every day, and to pick up and return his daughters to afterschool care or to his ex-wife's place.

During our first two years of marriage, Jeff stripped me of at least $35,000, and my expenses didn't stop there. I provided many things for Jeff's daughters throughout our marriage, including medical and dental insurance premiums for them through the company I worked for, plus co-payments when they visited the doctor or dentist. I bought them new eyeglasses because they had not had an eye exam or new glasses for four years, and were initially still wearing the pair of glasses they had in first grade, and every year, I provided eye exams and glasses. I made sure they got their hair cut regularly. They had never before gone to a salon and had their hair cut by a professional. On a regular basis, I bought them clothes and items necessary to take care of their personal hygiene. I paid for their afterschool care when it was not paid by Jeff's ex-wife. Lindsey and Laura attended a Catholic grade school, and Jeff's ex-wife paid their tuition for the first three years of our marriage. After the first three years, I ended up financing their Catholic education until they attended a public school for their senior year of high school.

Throughout our marriage, and especially when it ended, I was angry and resentful about how much I had given financially to Jeff and his daughters. I had allowed all three of them to suck my savings and mutual funds dry. I have *never* gotten over that anger, and now that Jeff is dead, my anger about the high cost of marrying him is more intense than ever. It's the only thing I can think about. I have always been fiercely annoyed at Lindsey and Laura for two reasons: (1) paying for their needs took away from what I could have provided for the whole family; and (2) I view them as the main reason why Jeff was always so angry, and the times when Jeff was angry put the greatest stress on our marriage.

By marrying Jeff, I *voluntarily* made a commitment to love him no matter what his health or financial situation would be. But I never adopted his daughters. Out of the three adults in the picture—Jeff, me, and his ex-wife—I should have been the last one to be financially responsible for them. His ex-wife—their mother—should have been first, and she should have used Jeff's support money to pay for their expenses. The amount of money I paid for tuition was ridiculous. I always viewed it as a needless expense, and because Nicole attended a public school, I felt that she was never given an equal share of my money.

When Jeff's ex-wife stopped paying tuition, I asked Jeff to hire an attorney to get his divorce decree modified. His child support payments needed to be eliminated because I had been paying for all of their daughter's expenses, and I had receipts to back up my claim. I also wanted his ex-wife to pay tuition or have them attend a public school, which would not have required any legal intervention because tuition costs were not mentioned in his divorce decree. For the first six years of our marriage, Jeff allowed his ex-wife to ignore the expenses she was responsible for. He paid child support, and let her use it as supplemental income for her own needs. When he finally hired an attorney, it took a year and a half after that to get his ex-wife's signature on an amended divorce decree. I was furious that it took so long! Jeff *never* pushed his attorney for action, and he never hired an attorney willing to force any action from his ex-wife's side. Jeff blamed the year-and-half delay for an amended decree on his ex-wife's refusal to sign the documents. But I blamed it on his attorney's lack of decisive action. Jeff allowed his attorney to ignore deadline after deadline for her signature. I never understood how she got away with ignoring all of the requests to sign an amended decree. Why wasn't there *one* cut-off date set for her to sign? If she didn't sign by the set date, then his attorney should have set up court mediation. Lindsey and Laura were 17 years old when Jeff's ex-wife agreed to no child support, and that she would pay their tuition. By that time, they had only one year of high school remaining and attended a public school for their senior year. Go figure!

The Mr. Hyde Side of Jeff

As I mentioned previously, Jeff's inability to hear adequately caused him to be paranoid. His hearing was so poor that at a restaurant, when the waitress asked what kind of salad dressing he wanted, he would answer with baked potato toppings. Jeff always thought that other people (mainly me) were whispering about him and undermining his intelligence, decisions, and his ability to be a parent. He would lash out at me and accuse me of conspiring against him with Lindsey, Laura, Nicole, and even with his family. His ongoing belief that I was scheming against him always left me dumbfounded.

I convinced Jeff to see a hearing specialist—and the specialist was confident that surgery could correct his type of hearing loss. Unfortunately, the surgery failed to improve his hearing. The next step was hearing aids. Jeff agreed that hearing aids were badly needed. He tried them for a week and refused to wear them after that because they "squealed" in his ears. He never went back for a consultation or an adjustment. As a result, his hearing loss continued to make him paranoid and continued to be a major source of his anger.

When Lindsey and Laura were around, the amount of alcohol Jeff drank increased and his anger quadrupled. When he drank, he would get furious at the simplest things. Everything boiled down to our apparent lack of respect for Jeff—he let us know by pointing out dirt, scuff marks, and food on the kitchen floor, or crumbs on the kitchen countertop. He also pointed out when only one Pop-Tart was taken from the 2-pack, the cookie package was left open on the counter, or the cereal box wasn't sealed and closed. It irritated him that the kids "stabbed" the peanut butter with a knife instead of swiping it to make it look smooth. We never ate dinner as a family at the dining room table, and that wasn't because the kids were involved in so many extra-curricular activities that we had to juggle schedules. It was because Jeff couldn't stand to watch the kids eat. He said their manners were disgusting and he couldn't stand how they got food all over their sleeves, and talked with their mouths filled with food.

Jeff always said that it didn't matter who didn't flush the toilet, who left the granola bar box open, or who didn't screw the milk lid on tight. We were all supposed to cover each other's asses, and it didn't matter if one of us was doing more work than another. As a result, I was constantly scouring the refrigerator, pantry, and countertops for items that weren't sealed and put away. I endlessly wiped the kitchen countertops and floor and picked up crayons, Barbies, puzzles, and school books before he saw that any of the kids had abandoned their items for a few minutes while they went to the bathroom. I spent an enormous amount of time trying to keep the kids out of Jeff's face, and protecting all of us from his outbursts.

No matter how much effort I put into covering all of our asses, there was always something I missed. Jeff would explode and tell us how much he sacrificed, and how ungrateful we all were for everything he did for us. Jeff used the word "fuck" a lot. We constantly heard, "Fuck all of you for disrespecting me. I fucking provide you with every fucking thing, and you can't even show me any fucking respect."

Jeff's anger was never expressed in an understandable way. If he had just discovered a backpack on the couch before Lindsey and Laura asked what was for dinner, his response to the dinner question was "Have I ever not provided you with dinner? I provide you with dinner every fucking night." That was supposed to translate into, "Take your backpack upstairs to your bedroom." When he was sweeping the kitchen floor and one of the kids said, "I'm hungry," his response was, "How the fuck does that identify who you are?" He really meant, "While I'm sweeping the floor of stuff from the bottom of your shoes, go pick up Barbie and her clothes from the living room floor, and the dog needs to go outside."

Jeff's reactions to everyday occurrences caused Nicole and me to walk on eggshells all the time. Nicole learned to avoid Jeff when she saw beer cans stacked up on the kitchen steps, but Lindsey and Laura didn't react the same way. They never avoided Jeff and would constantly seek him out to give him a hug. Lindsey and Laura had (and still have) an obsessive need to hug people. They wanted a hug from Nicole and me every time they saw us, whether it was three minutes after a hug or three hours after a hug. Their need for a hug from Jeff was *incessant* and they would hug him constantly. In response to Jeff's outbursts and anger at the lack of respect for him, Lindsey and Laura would hug him and say, "Ooooooh, I'm reeeally sorry, Dad!" Then they would say "I love you" as a question, expecting and needing to hear "I love you" back. Nicole and I didn't like the hugs and *I love you*s. Jeff HATED them. Jeff always took a step backward when he saw that his daughters were going to hug him, so Nicole and I called their hugs with Jeff "hang-on-hugs." They needed to hang on to him while hugging him because he was always trying to move away. Every time they saw Jeff, they went through the hang-on-hug and *I love you* routine again, which pissed him off even more.

Often, after spending hours at the neighbors' house, drinking outside on the lawn until midnight, Jeff would come home in a drunken stupor and get angry at me. He would grab my shoulders and shove me down on the kitchen floor. One time, my knees were so bruised that when I went to the doctor's office for my annual checkup a week later, my doctor asked about the bruises. (I told her that I fell on the ice.) Other times, when Jeff came home in the same state of mind, I would walk away and go into the bedroom. That infuriated him. He would come after me and put his hands around my neck and shake my head, all the while saying, "Fuck you, fuck you, fuck you."

Coping: Nicole is the one who understands Jeff and my relationship the best. I had forgotten some of the things that Nicole has remembered, like the time Jeff threw an ashtray through the window, shattering the glass everywhere. Nicole understands that I'm grieving the relationship that I feel I *should have had* with Jeff. We both loved the amazing man Jeff was capable of being, but there's no sugar-coating the person that he was a lot of the time. Nicole helps me laugh at Jeff's idiosyncrasies. She will grab ice cream from the freezer and eat the ice cream right from the carton and say, "I'm doing this just to piss Jeff off."

Jeff continuously expressed anger about his ex-wife, and I think sometimes he hated his daughters because she was their mother. I think they were a constant reminder of his ex-wife because they have many of her personality traits. When they were around, his anger was so much more intense, that it made me *hate* the times they were with us.

Jeff's divorce decree did not list days, times, or holidays when his daughters would be with each parent. It didn't specify who would pay for day-to-day expenses, such as school supplies, afterschool care, or haircuts. Medical expenses and tuition were also not mentioned in the divorce decree. The only expense the divorce decree mentioned was the amount Jeff would pay to his ex-wife for child support.

As a result, his ex-wife picked up their daughters and dropped them off at our place whenever it was convenient for her. They were there after school, for dinner, and overnight whenever she decided they would be there. If they were wearing the clothes I had bought for them when his ex-wife picked them up, I never saw those clothes again. When I asked Lindsey and Laura to bring back some clothes so that they could have clean clothes the next time they were with us, they told me they couldn't find them at their mom's place. Jeff would shrug his shoulders, roll his eyes, and walk out of the room.

Jeff's ex-wife frequently forgot to pick up their daughters, and they would call Jeff for a ride. It angered Jeff (and rightfully so) that his ex-wife was so negligent. However, after picking them up and taking them where they needed to be, he came home angry and took out his frustration and lack of control he felt regarding his ex-wife on me. It was as if I was living in his ex-wife's shadow—he would begin to see me as if I were her. It always turned out to be *my lack of concern* for his daughters that caused him to pick up the slack and be "solely responsible" for them all the time.

Jeff never set boundaries for Lindsey and Laura, and they never had any type of routine, such as a scheduled bedtime. Often, they would come to our place after school, sleep on the couch well into the evening, stay up until the wee hours of the morning, and attend school the next day. While they were sleeping on the couch, Nicole and I were expected to walk and talk softly so as to not to disturb them. If I suggested they go up and sleep in their own bedrooms, or better yet, have a more routine sleep schedule, Jeff chided me, saying that it was their mom's fault that they needed to sleep at odd times of the day. Jeff said that his ex-wife was bipolar, sleeping for days at a time or hitting mania episodes when she would function on little sleep for a week or so. According to Jeff, since his ex-wife never had a normal sleep schedule, their daughters *had a right* to "regulate" their sleep time.

If I ever asked Lindsey and Laura to do something, like take out the trash, wipe the counter tops, pick up their things etc., Jeff told me I was insulting their intelligence and intentionally demeaning them. He would defend their lack of knowledge as being his ex-wife's fault. As a result, they were never responsible for themselves or their personal things, and never did chores around the house. I eventually came to view them as vampires of my energy because of the time I spent doing their laundry, flushing their toilet, wiping their hair from the sink, emptying their trash, picking up after them, transporting them, and covering their asses so their dad wouldn't be so angry when they were around. I guess it should not be a surprise that today, Lindsey and Laura are 25 years old and neither one of them has a driver's license.

The Dr. Jekyll Side of Jeff

When his daughters weren't around, Jeff would talk to Nicole about all kinds of subjects; the sky was the limit on the feelings and ideas they shared. Jeff was so much more than her biological father—she saw him every day from age 6 to age 14 and again during her first year of community college when she was 18 and 19 years of age. I traveled often for my job, and Nicole has always said that she loved the times when it was just she and Jeff together. When no one else was around, Nicole saw Jeff as a kind and compassionate father who made her feel safe. They communicated on a unique level, and Nicole has always said that she felt a special ability to connect with Jeff, as if they had known each other in a previous life.

When Jeff's father was diagnosed with cancer, he and each of his siblings stayed one night of the week with his mom and dad. Saturday nights were not covered by anyone, so Nicole and I stayed with his mom and dad every Saturday night until his father's death eight months later. Jeff was so grateful to us for that. His father's struggle and eventual death brought us closer together. We both learned that death is an important part of life, and we were thankful that we had the time to say goodbye to his dad.

Jeff had long hair that reached below the middle of his back. When he decided to have it cut, the hairdresser cut off a 14-inch braid and Jeff donated it to Locks of Love, a charity that uses donated ponytails to provide quality hair prosthetics to financially disadvantaged children suffering from hair loss.[2] After the 2001 murder of seven people, including five children, in Sioux City, Jeff felt very sad for the children. He bought a teddy bear over his lunch hour and stopped by the family's house to put it outside among the other tributes to the family that were already there. Jeff had some EMT training, and was one of the first civilian responders after a horrific plane crash in Sioux City that left 111 fatalities and 172 injuries. Jeff said that the crash scene was described by one Vietnam veteran he worked closely with at the scene as "a complete warzone." He received recognition and an award from the city for his outstanding service during the crisis.

After our divorce was final, Jeff wrote me a long letter and admitted that he alone was responsible for his actions during our marriage. He apologized for the many times he had hurt me, and took responsibility for making my life difficult—and sometimes unbearable. He said that he had been spending a lot

---

2   http://locksoflove.org/

of time evaluating what was important to him in his life, and that he was going through some painful self-analysis in order to understand his personal philosophies, beliefs, and virtues. He said he wanted to become a better person for both Nicole and me. He told me that he had always loved and cherished me, and that he could not possibly love anyone else more than he did me. The last part of his letter said he would be there for Nicole and me at any point in time if we needed him.

I shredded the letter, angry at him because of how hard I had tried, over and over again, to get his attention and work on our marriage. I was frustrated that he was just beginning to become aware of the misery he put me through, and I didn't believe that he realized how much damage he had actually done to my spirit. When I left Jeff, I felt like a shell of a person. I loved him, but he took everything from me.

My Struggle with Jeff and Mary as a Couple

The comments left by Mary's friends on Jeff's online obituary irked me no end. One condolence said that Mary's face lit up whenever she talked about Jeff. One friend said she was so happy that Mary had found Jeff to complete her life. My "favorite" condolence was, "[I] was always so genuinely heartened by seeing how happy and contented they appeared whenever one saw them. And how willing to embrace life together ... " It irritates and infuriates me that Jeff and Mary are being viewed together as a couple. Mary didn't even know Jeff very well. She had known him in high school 30 years ago, but they never even had the same group of friends there. Mary and her friends don't have a clue about the dominant Mr. Hyde part of Jeff's personality. Mary had a year and a half with Jeff. I had ten years with Mr. Hyde, aka Jeff, and he wore me ragged.

I went to hell and back every day, only to be sent back to hell the next day.

Coping: Nicole has helped me sort out my frustration about Jeff and Mary being viewed as a couple. As much as I didn't want to hear it, Nicole reminded me that when I left Jeff, I opened the door for him to have a relationship with someone else. If Jeff treated another family, or even his own family, better than he did us, it was a result of what he learned from us. After we left, Jeff realized how much had been taken away from him.

Coping: I have come to the conclusion, and allowed myself to accept, that Jeff was two different people. One side of Jeff was compassionate and caring, but the side I saw most often was mean and sometimes abusive.

Lindsey and Laura put together Jeff's obituary, and I'm feeling a tremendous amount of anger towards them for what they wrote. It infuriates me that they remembered their father as a saint. Their description of him is what they *wanted him to be* rather what he *was actually like*. They described him as "a loving and supportive father who enjoyed nothing more than spending quality time doing everything from T-ball to homework with his twin daughters, Lindsey and Laura. He had a wonderful and unique sense of humor. They laughed constantly ... We will miss his smile, laugh, sense of humor ... hugs, kisses, kindness, and good nature."

My reaction to that description of Jeff is, "WOW! Fucking-A! You've GOT to be kidding me!" Jeff NEVER spent quality time with his daughters—for Christ's sake, we never even ate dinner together. I struggled daily with the demons inside Jeff that apparently they never saw. How did that happen? I must have done one hell of a good job at shielding his anger from them. Jeff HATED hugs and kisses from his daughters, and it pissed him off when they would constantly hug EVERYONE. Jeff said his ex-wife was always giving hugs and saying "I love you" to everyone. When they acted like their mom, it absolutely put him over the edge.

> **Coping:** If this is Lindsey and Laura's initial grief coming through, then I guess I have to accept it and realize that there are few, if any, obituaries ever written that eulogize a person as a complete jerk.

> **Coping:** In my heart I know that Lindsey and Laura caused a lot of Jeff's anger because they were a constant reminder of his ex-wife. The fact that they never saw his anger, or never saw themselves as the cause of his anger, doesn't matter now. It bothers me that Mary never saw Jeff's true colors—she never lived with Jeff and his daughters as I did, but that doesn't matter now either. Jeff is dead, and Lindsey and Laura won't be pissing him off anymore.

When Jeff and I separated, we lived in different states. I wanted Jeff to sell the house (because I wanted my share of the money the house was worth) so, before I left, I listed the house with a realtor. Jeff got one offer that was not acceptable to him, and he never made a counter-offer. The realtor I hired eventually got fed up with Jeff, and told me that Jeff really didn't want to sell the house.

My divorce attorney was licensed in the state where I am living now, and was unable to legally handle the separation of property in a different state. I ended up giving Jeff the house and its contents free and clear. Jeff needed to get the mortgage under his name. That was easy because during our marriage, I made sure that all of our bills were paid and he now had an excellent credit rating. It was only paperwork that needed to be filed with the mortgage company. Since I was not "selling" the house to Jeff, he did not need a down payment or to pay for mortgage points and closing costs.

Several months before our divorce was final, Jeff lost his job and was out of work for over a year. During that time, his brother called me and asked if I thought Jeff might be taking money out of their 79-year-old mother's bank account. He and the rest of Jeff's family had noticed that a large sum of money had been withdrawn from the account. A week after I talked to Jeff's brother, his mom passed away. I honestly don't know if Jeff was using his mom's money to make mortgage payments during the time he was unemployed.

Eventually, Jeff found another job, but apparently not a job where he earned enough to continue to pay the mortgage. The house was foreclosed on and Jeff moved in with Mary sometime in 2011.

In Jeff's obituary, Lindsey and Laura wrote, "Jeff was sharing a home and his life with friend and partner Mary. She is very genuine, loving, and warm, and shares Jeff's sense of humor. Their relationship is very important and fostered personal growth, happiness, and fulfillment for Jeff. Mary's love is a tremendous, invaluable gift to both Jeff and his daughters. Thank you, Mary."

My reaction to that is, "Are you fucking serious, guys? I would like to smear fucking shit all over your faces." First of all, the description of Mary's personality traits in *Jeff's* obituary is completely out of line. We are remembering Jeff, not Mary. Secondly, if Jeff left this world as a better person, and had recently experienced personal growth, it certainly wasn't because of Mary. *I am the one* who gave Jeff a wake-up call. It's the soul searching he did too late in OUR relationship that made him work on his issues, and perhaps emerge as a better person. Mary found a man who had lost family because of his anger and alcoholism, who was unable to support himself or his daughters because he never had a decent paying job, and never took action to improve his life. When Jeff moved in with Mary, he probably realized that unless he found someone to provide him with a place to live soon, he would end up living in a cardboard box under a downtown bridge in Sioux City. Just in the nick of time, Jeff was lucky enough to find someone as stupid as I was to support him. What a charmer!

I suppose if you look at it that way, then his daughters are right—Mary's love was an "invaluable gift to Jeff"—an invaluable gift called a fucking place to live.

Coping: I know somewhere in the logical part of my brain that the comments about Jeff and Mary's relationship in his obituary were not written to spite me. But my emotional side refuses to merge with my logical side, so their viewpoint of Mary giving them a tremendous and invaluable gift makes me want to scream! They spent little time with Mary compared to the time they spent with me. I want to say, "Please, go to Mary and suck an equal amount of money and energy from her that I experienced. Then let's evaluate how she feels about you guys."

Mary's love was *short-term*. Jeff and I had a commitment together called *marriage*, not a year-and-a-half relationship. I tried desperately to keep our marriage together despite everything that was taken from me. After pondering over the section of his obituary describing Mary and Jeff's relationship, I keep thinking that if Jeff had not been busy fostering "personal growth, happiness, and fulfillment" with his "friend and partner," then he might be alive today.

> **Coping:** Who knows what Mary and Jeff's future would have been? Maybe it would have been a long, lasting, and loving relationship, or it might have been that Mary would have ended up leaving Jeff for the same reasons I did. And maybe she would have ended up giving her house to Jeff too. The bottom line is that Jeff and Mary's future together is moot. They will definitely not have a relationship together now.

The brutality of Jeff's murder has been especially difficult for me. He was bludgeoned with a crowbar while sleeping on the couch we picked out together when we were married. I slept on that couch when Jeff snored and I couldn't go to sleep next to him, or when Jeff was so drunk that I didn't want to sleep next to him. Jeff and I watched movies, *Saturday Night Live*, Comedy Central, and college football games while sitting on that couch together. Much to Jeff's disapproval, that couch was Nicole's primary play area. It sickens me to know that couch was the scene of such a brutal murder.

My mind goes wild as I imagine what the crime scene must have looked like. Jeff's brother told me that, although Jeff's heart was still beating when he arrived at the hospital, it stopped before any type of surgery could be performed. The surgeon told Jeff's brother that even if Jeff's heart hadn't stopped, there were not enough pieces of Jeff's skull available to put it back together (even with artificial skull plates), and several fragments of bone could possibly have been embedded deep inside Jeff's brain tissue.

I am haunted daily by the fact that Jeff was *murdered*. It seems that everywhere I look, there is a young man with red hair who looks identical to the ex-boyfriend as his face appeared in his arresting mugshot. There also seems to always be a truck identical to the one Jeff drove everywhere I look. Nighttime is the most difficult. My dreams have been horrific nightmares with crowbars, knives, and garden tools, and the ex-boyfriend's face behind all of those weapons. My nightmares include lots of blood, chunks of brain and skull parts on the walls, ceiling, carpet, picture frames, lamps, and end tables. My dreams include endless chases where either Nicole or I are trying desperately to get away from someone. When I wake up, my heart is racing and I'm gasping for air.

I have coped with my nightmares by sharing them with Nicole. She is haunted during the day with the same things I am experiencing and having the same type of nightmares. It has helped a tremendous amount to tell her my stories and listen to hers. We are finding validation through each other as well as some consolation that we are not going crazy.

I have also been documenting my dreams. I have frequently recorded my dreams throughout my life, so I'm comfortable grabbing my pen and dream journal to write what I remember when I wake. I continue to work with my dream journal throughout the day because usually, as the day goes by, I remember parts of my dreams that escaped me when I first woke up. I add what I remember throughout the day to my initial document. Reviewing my dream documents helps me pinpoint the particular aspects of Jeff's murder that I'm struggling with most. I have a long road ahead of me, yet I believe that recording and reviewing my dreams while awake is a good first step in getting my unconscious thoughts under control.

Nicole had the opportunity to view Jeff's body before he was cremated. The funeral home gave each member of Jeff's family (Jeff and his family had always considered Nicole as his daughter) time alone with Jeff's body to say their personal goodbyes. One of the first things Nicole told me that she said out loud to Jeff when seeing him was, "I hope you have finally found the peace that you were searching for during your life on earth." Ironically, that is one of the first thoughts I had about Jeff as well. I made a silent prayer to Jeff and told him those exact same words.

It has been two months since Jeff's death, and I'm just beginning to let some of my anger loosen its restrictive grip on my heart. For me, because Jeff is dead, my anger towards him feels more a part of my past than my present. Viewing the anger as a part of my past has allowed me to let it go more easily than if I were still in the midst of the anger. I'm focusing on what I have learned from my relationship with Jeff that can help me push forward to my future. There will *never* be an easy way around my anger; the only constructive way is *through* the anger to emerge on the other side as a kinder, gentler, and wiser person.

When I feel my anger toward Jeff rear its head, it helps if I stop myself and try to pinpoint exactly *what* I am angry about. I don't allow myself to be angry in general terms. I refuse to allow myself to say, "Jeff treated me like shit." I force myself to be specific and say, for example, "It sucked so badly when I felt I was living in his ex-wife's shadow, and he blamed me for the things *she* was doing to him." I am determined to define what I can learn from being treated that way. I have the opportunity to accept the challenge, recognize Jeff's behavior, and not allow myself to walk in anyone's shadow again. That is so simple to write! Yet *it is work*, and resolving my anger will be a work in progress for some time. But I know I can do it.

The key for me in resolving my anger towards Lindsey and Laura is to look at Jeff's and my relationship from their viewpoint. How would they ever know how much they and Jeff took from me emotionally and financially? The obituary they wrote that included so much about Mary has nothing to do with me. As with my anger towards Jeff, I'm moving forward and recognizing the past as exactly that—the *past*. Yes, I gave a lot, but it's over and it's time to move forward.

The true grief from Jeff's death that I will feel forever is for Nicole. His death has cut her heart deeply. Nicole has never sugar-coated the Mr. Hyde side of Jeff, yet she has been able to take the high road over the intense anger that I express about Jeff. Nicole has so much appreciation for having had Jeff in her life. She experienced him as a remarkable gift, and felt that fate could not have chosen a better person to be her father.

Listening to Nicole talk now that Jeff is dead has been extraordinary. I had never realized how close they were, and Nicole admits that even she didn't realize how much they shared until after his death. Nicole has softened my anger. She knew Jeff in a very special way, and he gave her so much of what I think of as her spirit. How can I be angry at Jeff for that? I'm learning to appreciate all that he gave to my daughter.

Allowing myself to be angry and focusing on redirecting that anger to benefit my life now has been important in returning to a normal, and hopefully improved, state of mind since Jeff's death. I am blessed to have a daughter who is willing to share with me her deep and personal relationship with Jeff. Nicole has helped me to overcome so much anger by allowing me to see Jeff through her eyes. Jeff as Dr. Jekyll had a positive influence in Nicole's life and I am grateful. I'm letting go of Mr. Hyde's emotional hold on me—may he rest in peace!

CHAPTER 10

IT SEEMED CRAZY BECAUSE IT WAS

~ CAROL WHEELER ~

[Editor's Note: The writer met her soon-to-be-husband when he was an associate editor at Life *magazine, probably among the most glamorous of professions in the early 1960s. Sixteen years later, after marriage and a son who was then 9, the husband, now a university teacher, lost his marbles (not to put too fine a point on it) completely and was in and out of institutions from then on. They divorced, and about 17 years after they parted, the writer met her second husband, who died suddenly after they had shared almost four years together. Her first husband has also since died.]*

Oh, how happy I was when we finally called it quits. But that doesn't begin to tell the story of our married life, which was perfectly acceptable, even very happy, until the day almost 15 years after our wedding, when he insisted I stop using his late father's bureau (an antique which I had beautifully restored) for my clothes, in our bedroom.

I'm afraid my response (we were in bed—it was nighttime) was along the lines of "Are you crazy?" I'd just spent hundreds of dollars on the restoration. I'd just carefully arranged all of my lingerie, shirts, sweaters—all of it—in drawers I'd lined with pretty paper. I'd even asked him weeks ago if the object, its use, and its placement would bother him, and he'd assured me it wouldn't. So it did seem crazy.

And it was. That was the beginning of a nightmare that lasted for a few decades and wasn't really over until he died in a nursing home for old crazy people. In between, there were many bizarre events, including the regular fits that forced him to leave his classroom (he taught at a city university campus) and go pretty much straight to the hospital. There was the time, years later, when our son, Nicholas, had to break into his apartment to get him to the hospital, but that's another story, and it belongs to Nicholas.

When it all began, we had been about to leave New York for a year. Tom was going on sabbatical from his regular teaching job—he'd found a new job teaching in Paris. Nick was enrolled in the American School there. We had found a year's rental in the 16th *arrondisement* and subleased our own co-op apartment in New York to a French diplomatic family. All those plans of course went into the shredder (as I rather felt I had, ultimately). For the next year, everyone I faintly knew, if they saw me on the street, said, "But I thought you were going to Paris." Nick went back to his old school, which I know wasn't easy, and of course, got the same questions. So it turned out to be pretty painful— going from what was promised to be heaven (a year in Paris!) to a hell (staying at home with everything changed for the worse) that I never realized existed.

The no-turning-back events began a few months after the bureau incident (which had culminated in my buying a new one and having someone else take the first one away) one summer weekend in the Berkshires. By then, it was becoming clear that all of our wonderful plans were not going to work, but I was still in denial. A colleague of Tom's was visiting with his wife, and Tom was behaving so strangely (I don't exactly remember in what way—time does, thankfully, draw a veil) that I had to ask them to leave. (They got it.) I then gathered some stuff, and our son, and drove off, back to the city, as we seemed to be of no use to Tom, and he was hurting us emotionally, very painfully. (At the time, he was seeing a psychoanalyst in town, but didn't have an appointment for a few days.)

When I got back to our apartment (it was the first time ever that I had driven back to New York in traffic), I called him. We talked about how he was feeling, how he needed to relax and come in the next day. But on the next day, hearing nothing, I called again. *Ring, ring, ring* and on and on it went, until finally (there were no answering machines then), he picked up, sounding thick-voiced, almost stupefied.

"The pain," he said. "I took some pills to stop the pain." I told him I would call someone and hung up, in tears (as I am now, writing this). I hugged Nicholas, looked at him, feared for him, and called some friends who lived nearby. They said they would go and see what was happening. Luckily, our supply of pills was very meager—mostly aspirin I think, but he did take a great deal. The next day, I arranged for our son to have a playdate, and I drove back up to our house in the beautiful, verdant countryside, basking unaware in the July sun.

Our friends had taken Tom to what we all thought of as the best local hospital. The hospital had pumped his stomach (that classic phrase—I think that's really what they called it), and there he was, off-kilter as ever, deeply depressed, but alive, wearing shorts, which seemed the greatest indignity. The doctor explained that they didn't have the facilities to treat mental illness there, but he had worked the phones and managed to get a place for Tom at Payne Whitney, a division of New York Hospital, which seemed a great coup at the time (but not for much longer). When I decided to drive him down there the next day, I didn't realize that I was entering the maw of the Great Mental Illness Machine—a maw from which there would be no turning back, ever. *Abandon hope, all ye who enter here* could have been written over the door—not for everyone, maybe—but for me. And for Tom.

When we arrived in New York City that day, after a hair-raising drive on the freeway, during which I was sure Tom would open his door on the passenger side and just slip out onto the road, our first red light on our way to Payne Whitney across town was at 96th Street and Central Park West. Who should be crossing the road, but my very own psychiatrist! I resisted honking, but I am sure I could have used his help.

By the time a few years had passed, Tom had been an inmate of just about every mental wing of every New York City (and its suburbs) hospital. Every time, he'd leave the hospital somewhat better (not the hospital, him, although never *all* better), and then stop the medication within a few weeks, and slowly, inexorably resume the madness. When I think of it now— the torture he had to endure—I can and do weep. At the time, I thought only of the torture *I* was enduring—I took a valium every single night for an entire year to go to sleep—I, who had never taken a sleeping pill or anything but an aspirin in my life. I came to love valium more than anything in the world, except for our son. I still know, and firmly believe that throughout, it was way more painful for me and for Nicholas—Tom didn't quite get what was happening, after all. Much of the time, he thought he was perfectly fine—as when it all culminated in a public display.

We were walking down Broadway to the theatre one summer night, after it had all happened—the overdose, Payne Whitney, my winter trip to the Yucatan with Nicholas (Tom wouldn't go), his refusal to see a doctor regularly, and he began muttering loudly, "They'll find out." He went on that way when we got on the bus. I was mortified. What he meant, I was pretty sure at the time (mainly because he'd talked about it before), was that when his book was published, "they"—the world in general? His college? (Harvard, of course.) The publishers?—would know he was actually a fraud.

He really wasn't a fraud, and no one would ever have thought so. His book was about teaching disadvantaged college students to write—*The Great American Writing Block*, it was called—and it was interesting and relevant enough to be featured in a review in the Sunday *New York Times Book Review* on the same Sunday that it was excerpted in the *New York Times* magazine. Phil Donahue (who had a rather literary TV talk show at the time) called right after that. By then, Tom was in a locked ward.

The first time that happened (the Payne Whitney time), I prayed for his recovery. Well, the kind of praying atheists do, anyway. But after a while, it was clear that, since Tom refused to recognize that there was anything wrong, there was no chance of recovery. I went with him to one new doctor whose office he stormed out of because the doctor confirmed that he was sick and needed treatment. The analyst he'd been going to before his total breakdown was completely out of the picture. This analyst had been so shocked that Tom tried to kill himself that he'd submitted his bill before the end of the month. Just in case, I guess.

Once, at that same general point, Nick was near a window, and Tom did try to, well, almost, push him out (I find it's still difficult to be totally categorical about what really happened).

We lived on the ninth floor, overlooking Riverside Park and the George Washington Bridge. (The window they were standing at, however, was in the kitchen, and faced a narrow areaway—not that it matters.) On the other hand, Nick was only 9, so I suppose if Tom had really wanted to, he could have done it. It was a big window. I saw Tom take hold of Nick just above the elbows and push him toward the opening—in memory, I literally feel that push on my own arms. I intervened somehow, but it's a memory I cannot quite recreate because it's too horrible to dwell on. I don't know if Nick remembers it or even if he knew what was happening at the time. I hope not.

It was then that I realized that it had to be over. My own therapist counseled me to make a decision and stick to it. That's what I did. I knew I couldn't continue this way, so just a short time after the incident on Broadway, when we were out for a walk, I told Tom that he had to leave. He said he'd kill himself. I said, "That's your decision." Somehow that did it. He moved to the Harvard Club. But in a month or so, he found an apartment, and in another month, he went totally bonkers again. This time, it was just as I was starting a new job, and it was also August, the month when psychiatrists leave New York.

So it was me who had to go and get him and take him to the hospital again. I'll never forget the cab driver telling me to have a nice day. I didn't.

For all these reasons and more, I wished for my first husband's death for many years, and when it happened I was, well, by then I was numb. I'd just lost my second, much-adored husband to cancer, and I didn't really think I could feel much of anything anymore. It had taken me the better part of two decades to be open to a new husband. One difficulty was that it took years to get an actual divorce. Tom's own lawyer couldn't make him see reason, so even with a separation agreement, the actual legal divorce didn't happen until about ten years later.

Maybe, too, there was something in me that still realized how lucky I had originally been to find a man like Tom, despite the unhappy ending. Certainly, something prevented me from being interested in any other man for a very long while. I think it was more than just the raw pain of what had happened. From what I'd heard from other women, "good men really are hard to find," so until my incredibly beyond-good, tall, handsome, smart, witty, caring, sane Joe came along, it was easy enough to ignore the others.

A few years after both their deaths, however, I find that I am far from numb. Now I have two dead men to feel sad and nostalgic about. A widow only once, but being a... what? Remarried and re-widowed remnant of a former spouse? The fact that there's no word for it that I know of is also depressing.

The past has its hold on us, though not as irrevocably as we sometimes think. My more distant past with this man, my first husband, was all joy and delight, in my memory at least. Our first years together affected me deeply in the best ways possible (is everyone's first marriage like this?)—my face hurt sometimes from smiling too much, a disability I managed to cope with nicely. We were happy.

After we finally separated, there were horrible, vile, seemingly endless answering-machine messages that speared my heart and hurt my head to listen to—I had to listen to them privately, directly into my ear (I could feel the venom gushing in) to be sure our son (who was, of course, living with me, but still seeing Tom when possible) didn't hear. When the two of us still lived together with our son, it was worse, in a threatening, even frightening way. In fact, it was my fears for our child that made me insist on separation. (Well, not entirely, to be fair—I was also afraid for myself, physically and emotionally. But especially, I didn't see how I could be the mother to a little boy and nursemaid to a mental patient—an uncooperative one at that—at the same time.)

Nick had his own problems, but having a totally off-the-wall father was a big one that led to a lot of other little ones. Much later, when he was a teenager, he told me how hard it was to distinguish between his father's reality and the other, real reality. First, his father's was more dramatic, and I guess that might be appealing to a romantic child. Then of course, children do naturally believe their fathers, especially if they've originally been loving and stable and helpful and generous. Although, once when he was still a little boy, and I was reminding him how his dad had been before his breakdown, Nick said, "I don't *remember* what he was like." Well, he wailed, actually.

At the time, I never wanted to see Tom again. I wished him dead, quite frankly. It seemed death would be best for him, as well as the rest of us. But now that I cannot ever see him again alive, I begin to remember his kindness, his love, all that he gave to me and our son. My first ski trip, my first trip to Europe, my only child, my sense of myself as a desired woman, and desired by a man with two degrees from Harvard, from a family in the ruling class. To Nick, he gave himself as a very involved father, a beautiful early childhood, a house in the country with a hand-built tree house and a meadow for dreaming, a giant vegetable garden to weed and pick, a pony (quite large), and many wonderful father-son horseback rides in the country.

Of course, one reason I was determined NOT to see him was that the drugs he would only take when he was in the hospital gave him the jerky gait and contorted face of a person with tardive dyskinesia (despite the fact that he took far fewer than he should have), and I couldn't bear to see that in my once handsome, open-faced husband. Other reasons were his ingrained (yet low-key) arrogance, alternating with his complete denial (both personified by the fact that he would not take the drugs because how could there be anything wrong with HIM?).

Some of that arrogance was simply ingrained maleness, I always thought, and I'm sure a lot of it was simply the lack of insight that can come with mental illness. Yet I'm also sure that some of it was a direct result of his lifelong position in the upper-est of the American upper-class, with a Fortune 500 CEO for a father, and the granddaughter of a slave-holder for a mother, with sail-boating and garden-tending, swanky prep schools, and haughty club memberships all simply a given in his life. (Both of his parents were lovely people in most ways, and not snobby at all, but still ...). Possibly that newer word, "entitled," is a more appropriate description in this case. It seems to take the edge off that very cutting, sharp "arrogance" description. Although the label "entitlement" may have been invented to make the rich seem less haughty and cruel (it doesn't work for me, but I think it does for some), it may be quite right for the rather sweet man I married.

Tom, too, was anything but a snob. He went out of his way to be not just nice, but friendly to the servants (well, of course his family had servants). He taught disadvantaged kids at a college of the city university (and loved them, and wrote a book about them), where he worked after his two-decade stint as a correspondent and editor for *Life* magazine. After all, he married me, a little Jewish girl from the at-least-metaphorically "wrong" side of the tracks. He was an old-fashioned, kind of unbearably innocent liberal—despite the Harvard degrees—as was his father before him, of whom Senator Bill Benton (for whom Tom worked in his youthful, political phase) once said, "Look at your father, a huge success, and not very smart at all," or words to that effect.

In fact, the "to that effect" effect is one of the reasons I so miss my first husband, and have ever since we broke up. Even when he was alive and after we divorced, I couldn't just ask him what those words were exactly, not after the breakdown. He actually refused to speak to me at all for at least the last decade of his life, a rule I had to be grateful for at the time. But now, I weep knowing that this impasse will never be overcome. I will always want to talk to him about our shared past, our son, the words someone said to him once, whose cousin Cousin Mary Evelyn really was, how her granddaughter is related to our nephews—so much, and it will never be possible. His death ended all hope that it would ever be different. It's a hole at the heart of my life.

Two do live as one, do become one in some important ways, I now realize. No matter what breaks you apart, it can turn out to be a painful break, and one you will have to feel deeply eventually, even if you don't feel it right away. We were a couple for more than 16 years, and of course, as the parents of a child together, it goes on forever. Well, almost forever—now that he's dead, it's just me. Obviously, given the circumstances, our son has spent some time trying not to think about him. It's a big chunk of a life and it cannot be ignored.

In fact, our son was enormously gentle and kind to his father toward the end of his life. He visited his father in the institution where he lived, which was inconveniently located and probably not very comfortable for visitors (I never went there), and certainly not for Nick. When Tom died, Nick cared very much. He wasn't numb in the least. It was very different for him, as I tried to explain one night when he, Nick, was 9 years old, and I was telling him that Daddy was moving out. "It's true, Mom, I understand. It's not so bad for me—I don't have to sleep in the same bed with him," he said.

At the time, I tried to be understanding, to see my husband as "sick"—can't help it, no fault of his. But I couldn't do it. I hated him for what he did to us. From the depths of anger and sorrow, from the waves of sobbing that took over my life, I could summon no shred of sympathy for this man who had ruined our lives. I must add that his total denial of the fact that there was anything wrong with him made it particularly difficult to have any sympathy.

No doubt, I would never have become a magazine editor or writer if he hadn't fallen apart, but so what? I didn't need that. I liked being a wife and mother. I liked having a beautiful old house in the Berkshires for weekends and summers, and a spacious Upper West Side apartment with a drop-dead view of the George Washington Bridge in New York. I liked having time for everything. I liked puttering around the house, entertaining friends and relatives, and being part of, for quite a while, everyone's vision of a happy family. I liked the prospect of nothing ever really changing, dishonest as that thought might have been. I liked being envied. I hated being pitied, as it turned out. Maybe that was part of why I had none of that for him. But then he died. Alone, almost, in a nursing home. Our son was deeply affected, of course. I barely reacted, since I was still in pain over my second husband's death, which had occurred a month before 9/11, which I also barely noticed.

Now when something reminds me of Tom, I recall him fondly, without the pained bitterness of the past. A passage in an Umberto Eco novel, for instance: "With my mother, I spoke French ... when I speak it here in Paris, it sounds as if I've learned it in Grenoble, where the purest French is spoken ..." Grenoble is where Tom learned his quite fluent French. He spent a college year at the university there, before there was such a thing as The Year Abroad, and in Paris, he was sometimes taken for a French-speaking Swiss—rather brilliant for an American! I was so proud to be with him in those days.

The other day, I was reading something about peonies. When Tom was still alive (or even when he hadn't been dead for all that long), I would have moved on and not even wanted to read anything about that flower, which meant thinking about my ex-husband. He was an amazing gardener, and when we moved to that old farmhouse in the Berkshires (just for weekends and summers), he rescued all manner of flora from the confines of history. Peonies were among them. He discovered little shoots in the lawn and moved them to a bed right under the kitchen windows, cultivated them, watered them, and cared for them until we had big beautiful peony bushes every year. The flowers were a luscious shade of pink and they made the house beautiful, outside and in.

He found little traces of lilacs, too, and made a hedge down at the dirt road our house was on. That was an occasion for quoting Whitman: "When lilacs last in the dooryard bloomed," etc. and so on, and talking about why Whitman wrote it, and about Lincoln too. Just as the Fourth of July was an occasion for reading the Bill of Rights at lunch, not just for having hotdogs and potato salad. For various presidents' birthdays, we read aloud from their works. It was not the usual smug non-thinking American life that our child was born into, or that we lived.

As you can see, my first husband was quite well-grounded in literature and in history at the time when he was still capable of anything other than total self-absorption. Maybe his approach to everyday life and history is why everyone always assumes I have a college degree (in fact, I dropped out after a year). He gave me that way of looking at things too. That, and also the vegetable gardens in the country, which were, of course, prolific. We had everything—even our own corn! Corn picked fresh and immediately cooked was like nothing anyone had ever tasted before. All because of my now-dead ex-husband.

So now I miss Tom—really, oddly. When I daydream about my second husband, a man who helped me to understand, at long last, what love was all about, and who was the exact opposite of a mental patient (being a psychiatrist), Tom soon enters my daydreams too. Despite how different they were from each other, I loved them both, and they both loved me. I find myself wishing for both of them to be here. Joe, of course, always, but even Tom, if he could be the person he was before he lost his mind. I wasn't able to think of that before now; I didn't "remember what he was like," but now it's painfully clear. I chose him once. I would choose him again.

CHAPTER 11

REFLECTIONS OF AN EX-WIFE-TURNED-WIDOW

~ LAURIE WIMMER ~

Tom always said that he didn't want to go part by part. A diabetic with an unromantic view of life, he said that if ever the talk turned to amputation, I was to wheel him off a bridge. A good death, he said, was one that came all at once.

Well, he got his wish. A sudden, solitary cardiac event took him so abruptly that it nearly stopped the hearts of his many friends and admirers too.

Tom was a much-loved *bon vivant*. His quick wit, humble self-deprecating style, and undeniable good looks won the hearts of nearly everyone who met him, men and women alike. To be his wife was to play Gracie Allen to his George Burns.

I met Tom when he was serving in our state legislature. I was a lobbyist for our teacher's union. We partnered on a particularly contentious piece of education legislation; the long hours cemented a friendship that was as profound as our allegiance to the cause. Eventually, we moved in together and, two years later, we married. My 11-year-old son was Tom's best man and my 8-year-old daughter my maid of honor. His only child, a daughter, was a successful actress and lived in L.A.

with her manager. She faxed us a handwritten note of congratulations on the day of our wedding, but she never spent more than an hour or two in our home on the rare occasional visit–a fact that broke her father's heart.

Nonetheless, our lives were full and happy. We lived together for 11 years, raising my two children from a former marriage. We traveled, participated in public life, and shared a love for politics, history, literature, science, and the arts. Our many friends considered us a "power couple." Then Tom took a disability retirement from firefighting and became my house-husband. In addition to helping with the children, he began a room-by-room, long-term home remodeling project that remains unfinished to this day.

There was much laughter for most of those years, but sadness too. Tom's health challenges as a diabetic were only the beginning. There was the moment when I realized he was an alcoholic in need of treatment. I arranged a successful intervention with the help of friends, and he never touched another drop. But there was also the ever-present anger and self-loathing seething below the surface, the classic adult-child-of-an-alcoholic rage that he wouldn't address. He missed his beloved daughter. He seemed to have a death wish and gradually abandoned his healthful diet and exercise regimen. Twice in our marriage, he passed out in the middle of the night, heading toward a diabetic coma. It was the sound of his body dropping to the floor that awakened me and enabled me to save him both times.

An ex-football hero, he suffered one too many concussions, resulting in brain damage that mimicked attention-deficit disorder. Though he took medications for A.D.D. and depression, they didn't make much difference. Disordered thinking, lost concentration, inability to complete projects, overwhelming lethargy, occasional bitter rage, and what looked like a hoarding complex were qualities that made him feel like a classic underachiever, no matter how much he accomplished.

And Tom accomplished so much in his short life: Studentbody President in high school. Nationally recognized football star in college. Fire Captain and lobbyist for the State Firefighter Council. Service on state and city retirement boards. Union contract negotiator. Advocate for fire-safe cigarettes. Lifesaver. Hero. Father. Step-father. Friend. He even wrote a children's book about saving a cat stuck in a tree. Then there were the many times he came to the rescue of friends in trouble, offering intervention, counseling, friendship, and confidentiality when they found themselves in the grip of addiction.

On the home front, he offered my son, alienated from his biological father, a genuinely kind and worthy male role model. One particularly tough year, Tom persuaded me to let him homeschool Griffin to give him a break from the tortures of middle school. They concocted wild potions in our kitchen's "chemistry lab," experienced and studied September 2011 in real time, as scholars, and built model rockets to learn physics (which they subsequently treed in the park). My son learned from Tom's example that mirth and mind were as much a part of manhood as might and money.

Tom became my daughter's best playmate and co-conspirator in those years. He utterly spoiled her by granting her every wish. She never heard the word "no" to a request for his taxi service or expedition for treats. He made her afterschool snacks, told her that her butt should sue her skinny legs for "non-support," and generally made her laugh from morning to night. She adored her "Tommy." Even after our marriage ended, the two of them met monthly for a dinner or breakfast "gabfest," as he used to call them.

My children had never tasted soda pop or a donut before Tom's arrival on the scene, given my insistence on good nutrition. He was the lovable bad boy who could sneak candy into their lives and poke fun at their too-ordered mother. Though the children knew of Tom's sullen side, they rarely experienced it personally. For them, he was always at his absolute best.

One of the features of A.D.D. that bedeviled Tom was the habit of seizing on a focal point, obsessing about it, and then dropping it utterly when the interest passed—and the interest *always* passed. Every fad, every new product, every book or magazine that could capture his imagination was purchased and then, once the urge abated, was abandoned forever. He did this with things, and with people. Long-time friends were cherished, and then, suddenly, never seen again. Eventually, though I didn't see it coming, I became one of those objects of "hyperfocus," and then abandonment. Tom was a compassionate man, so when he lost interest in his first wife, and then in me, he never found a way to admit it outright. In each case, he simply set up the conditions for others to rearrange his life for him so that he could be free. That is how our marriage dissolved.

Tom "left me" long before I ended the marriage. Because he couldn't bear to hurt me with words, he did so with mean deeds. Though I suffered the hurts mostly in silence, I knew that something was seriously wrong. Tom refused to talk with me or a counselor. I feared that my options for relief were narrowing, but it took the intervention of friends to get me to leave him. Because of his serious health issues and impover-ished state (he would leave our home with just half a disability pension for income if we divorced), I was reluctant to end the marriage for fear that it would compromise his ability to stay healthy. Diabetes is an expensive lifestyle. In addition to that, I remembered vividly the nights he went down and would have died if he'd been alone. Divorce may be what he secretly craved, but it also promised to be a risky proposition. Finally, though, I told him that I couldn't go on any more. He was so relieved! Still, after his death, his daughter published a blog in which she claimed that it was his inability to pay for optimal health interventions that led to his death. In her thoughtful piece, she argued that President Obama's health care reform offered hope to those in her father's situation, though not in time to save him.

I used to joke that our dissolution was not so much a divorce as a "friendship-protection plan." Once the expec-tations of husbandhood were lifted from his shoulders, Tom became my best friend again. In the four years after we split up, we communicated weekly, sending each other arti-cles about the latest political outrage. We called each other frequently. He even made the occasional repair on my house. And, as he happily promised to do, he stayed close to my children and was involved in their lives. Two days before he died, he visited me to see the progress I'd made on a backyard landscaping project. Two days before that, he had me over to his new home to give me a tour. Though he eventually became involved with another companion, he never abandoned me as a close and treasured friend.

It was against this complicated history that I experienced his death. The new girlfriend did not call me. His father did not call me. His daughter did not call me. A mutual friend, who knew that I wouldn't learn of his passing from any of them, made the compassionate decision to reach out. Legal status notwithstanding, Tom was still the love of my life, and our friend knew that I had to be told. We should all be so lucky to have such friends!

The shock of the news led to numbness. I tend to go into disciplined autopilot when crisis demands it. I knew what to do, and I did it. I rushed to his 86-year-old father's side and helped him with those things that I could do best—writing (and paying a hefty bill for) his obituary, helping with some of his financial affairs, and offering my love and compassion. His father had now not only been predeceased by both of his sons, but was suddenly recast as the sole caregiver for his remaining child, a mentally disabled daughter. He and I discussed necessary details, and when Tom's daughter flew into town from the set of her latest movie, the three of us considered how best to honor Tom's memory and detangle his messy estate. I steeled myself for this work, and labored to resist crumbling in the agony of his loss.

Somewhere along the line, I was cut out of the planning and participation in Tom's memorial. Plans changed, other people were put in charge, sensitivities were hinted at, and in the end, my children and I were simply not a part of the final goodbye. One of Tom's childhood friends theorized that this was done to punish me for being the "other woman" when Tom's first marriage was ending. Fifteen years had passed since those days, but it may be a part of the explanation for what was a heartless exclusion masquerading as a "scheduling conflict."

I was a second wife, and ex-wife, and a step-mother—and somehow, our culture does not make room for such a person in life's ceremonial passages. The first wife attended the memorial. The new companion was also invited. I was the one intimate in this great man's life who was not to be present. My children, who loved their devoted second father, were also deemed inessential. In one of life's many small ironies, the two gentlemen who were asked to plan this exclusive wake were Republican stalwarts, deeply opposed to what I'm sure they would call "Obamacare"—not recognizing for a minute that universal health care access would have been their lost friend's salvation.

In a bizarrely twisted way, it was good that the small and exclusive send-off from which we were barred also left out many in public life who loved Tom and wanted to honor him one last time. I received dozens of letters and calls from political figures, close friends, and former colleagues, asking to be notified of his memorial. I soon realized that a man so large in life deserved more than one final honorary. That is how I ended up planning a Celebration of Life ceremony for Tom.

A lovely day in April set the stage for Tom's more public memorial service. His favorite music played in the background. A photographic album of his life, loves, and proudest accomplishments flashed on a screen over the crowd. All his favorite sweets—so dangerous to his health—were offered to attendees (he would have had it no other way). My son flew 3,000 miles from his college to be there. People from all aspects of Tom's life came from far and near to tell their funniest Tom stories. We created a list of "Tommyisms"—his wily quotations and one-liners–to help people honor him with laughter instead of tears. In the end, one fellow firefighter played bagpipes as other firefighters and guests lit brightly colored Chinese lanterns and sent them skyward as final celebratory offerings. Our hearts were made a bit less heavy by the camaraderie we shared. In giving these friends an outlet for their grief, my children and I had found one too. Though it was a wonderful and healing event, I still feel sharp pain whenever I permit myself to consider that Tom's daughter and father did not join us, nor did most of the attendees who had originally planned to be there, but were asked to be present for the first event instead.

If we as a species are to celebrate the best in humankind, we must be a part of making the world a better place. If we are to create beauty and love instead of poison and pain with our deeds, then there needs to be a rethinking of the treatment of ex-spouses in the aftermath of a loved one's death. We are more like in-laws than outlaws, but often, we are seen as inessential to the custom of mourning our dead. We may be overlooked and unnoticed, or aggressively excluded, depending on the circumstances, but we suffer no less than others in the orbit of the lost spouse. Graciousness is a rare commodity when one is focused on her own misery. I am sympathetic to the emotions that crowd out the ability one might otherwise have to be compassionate and thoughtful. It would seem that with a 50 percent divorce rate in our society, however, sheer humanity demands a reinvention of customs that focus on inclusiveness. If the circle of love is honored, it should be wide enough to include all who loved and were loved. The teachings of Emily Post should be revised to consider all broken hearts in these most difficult of human moments. In the absence of a contemporary protocol, I was forced to invent my own. Perhaps it may serve as a starting point in the reinvention of family grieving for others.

CHAPTER 12

Unexpected Consequences

~ Melanie ~

It was a phone call that I realized later I should have been prepared for, one that would come sooner or later, but found I wasn't.

My 26-year old was on the other side of the phone in Oklahoma City at approximately 9:00 p.m., with a sound in his voice I had never heard before. Quietly, as though very numb, he told me that his biological father had passed away. The funeral home, where his "father's" body had been taken, had notified him. The cause of death was "complications of multiple sclerosis." The funeral director had advised him that he needed to come and make financial arrangements with them since he was his son. My son was horrified.

I was speechless, of course. I had no idea how fast a complete memory can come rushing back and take no time to play out in my head. The memory took me back 26 years, very quickly! I was an unmarried teenager who had just given birth to a beautiful red-headed baby boy. I was 17 years old. I remembered how his father, a teenager himself, had come to the hospital the evening of his birth and denied him as his son. We never married, but to make understanding my story easier, I'll call him "my ex." We never had much of a relationship at all. We had met at a party, we had sex (lucky me, my first time!) that night and I became one of the teenage mother statistics of the mid-1970s. As young as I was, I was prepared to make a go of it with my baby boy all by myself. I barely had a relationship with my parents. Once I became pregnant, they cast me out of their lives. I had a baby out of wedlock. Doomsday for them—I had no other choice but to care for and love my son as best I could.

I snapped out of the time warp and reassured my son that his Dad and I would be on our way immediately. We would drive through the night to be at his side early the next morning. I told him we would help him through the entire experience. He was NOT alone. I say "his Dad" because a wonderful man came into my life when my son was 5 years old. My son carried my maiden name at that time. My husband adopted my son, uncontested after public notice in the newspaper where his biological father resided, when he was 8 years old. We had long wanted to make a formal adoption, yet I had allowed his biological father time to come around and face the fact that he had a son who looked just like him. Since that had not occurred, my son was adopted by this prince of a man. From 8 years old to his current 26 years, he had the best Dad a child could ever have wished for.

My son did not ever have the opportunity to meet his biological father face-to-face. He had spoken to him only once, over the phone—my son initiated the call when he was 19 years old and curious. We never withheld any names or circumstances of his birth from him. As he had grown older, I had told him more of the details, and so he knew what I knew about the person who provided the other half of the DNA to make him.

According to my son, the conversation had lasted over 2 hours. His biological father told my son that he knew he was his, but that since he was so young, and had no way to provide for him, nor marry his mother, he had chosen to stay out of his life. My son asked to meet him, yet that never happened, due to his biological father's choice. He had never married nor adopted any children. My son was his only child.

My son's biological grandmother had a very nasty personality. She let me know in no uncertain terms at the time she was told she had a grandchild that she wasn't old enough to be a grandmother, and therefore my son "couldn't be her son's child."

As my husband and I drove through the night, I didn't talk much about my son's early years, or the circumstances behind his creation and birth. Actually, I don't remember talking much at all for 11 hours: the time the drive took to get to my son. We would have flown, but there were no flights available. My motherly instincts told me that I would be at his side as quickly as I could get there, even if walking got me there faster.

When we arrived at my son's home, you could see the anxiety leave his face when he saw me. I knew we were close, but for one of the first times in my life, I realized what a good mother I was to my son. He knew he could count on me, and there I was—overnight, at his doorstep.

As we started to sit down and talk and find out how he was doing, he informed us that he had received a call from the funeral home that very morning to inform him that his father's family had notified them that "his son" would be paying for the funeral costs. (The "father's family" meaning my ex's mother.) The very one who had denied that my son was her grandson years ago was now "willing" to acknowledge his paternity to get out of paying for her own son's funeral! My son started to cry, saying he was just getting started in life and how in the world would he ever be able to pay for a $15,000 funeral? (My ex's mother had already picked out everything that *she* wanted for *her* son's funeral.)

Needless to say, my maternal tiger instincts instantly took over. Calmly, I told my son that we were there to help and make this process as smooth as possible. I also let him know that he would *not* be responsible for the funeral costs. I would see to it. I made up my mind that if my ex's mother wanted to make this tragic time ugly, well then, so be it.

I went in to another room and found the phone number for one of my ex's brothers. When I spoke with him (after extending my condolences, of course), I told him to get a message to his mother. IF she could come up with tangible legal proof that my son was her grandson—her recently deceased son's son—then he would be happy to pay for the entire funeral. Should she not have it, then back off!

Since my son didn't hear the conversation, I told him we would continue the day as planned. My son wanted to go to the funeral home to find out what they wanted from him exactly. When we arrived, we were met by the funeral director, who took us to a side office to talk. I explained that my son would not be paying for any of the funeral costs for someone that he did not know, did not have any relationship with, nor had my ex's family ever acknowledged that he even existed. The funeral director was stunned. You could tell that he expected us to discuss how my son would be paying for the deceased's funeral.

As I wanted to settle the matter once and for all for my son, I told the funeral director a little lie. I said that we needed to have swabs from the deceased's mouth in order to prove paternity and then determine who would be footing the bill. My son was shocked. I hadn't discussed this with him. I had discussed it with a geneticist friend of mine while on the drive to my son's house the night before. She had told me that the only thing you need from a deceased person is DNA and identification to prove paternity. You didn't need permission, court approval—nothing more. She told me that if I obtained the swabs, she would get the test done for me in her lab. She advised me to have the funeral director himself obtain the samples, then have the funeral home director specifically write out the details of where and from whom the samples were obtained. Being a nurse, I wrote everything out myself and had the funeral director sign and date the document after the swabs were obtained. Clean, cut, and dry.

I felt odd walking out of the funeral home with saliva samples from my ex in hand. Funny thing was that my son didn't seem to mind at all. He asked if we could stop and get something to eat on the way back to his house. He hadn't eaten anything since getting the phone call about his biological father's death the evening before. I thought, what the hell? We'll stop and eat. I have the samples stored the way they need to be. There's nothing stopping us from stopping to eat. No rush. We'll talk about what my son needs to talk about. We'll talk about ways we can help him through this—but other than that, we'd talk about how *our* family was doing.

My son expressed that he was so glad that his dad and mom were there to comfort him, as parents should always be. While we ate, my son asked me for the details about obtaining the DNA. He was worried that this would implicate him in paying for the funeral if it was determined, as he already knew, that my ex was indeed his biological DNA donor.

I told my son not to worry. I had only done it for him and him alone. I told him that my ex's family had no idea this specimen had been taken, and that he should have no worries about financial responsibility. We had *not* signed in when we entered the funeral home, nor did my son sign any paperwork of any kind while there. The Funeral Director obtained the specimen, but didn't have us sign anything for his own records to indicate that anything had transpired that day, or even make a copy of what I had him sign to indicate that *he* had obtained the samples from the deceased. It was the funeral director's word against ours. The Funeral Director had no way of proving that we were ever there, nor have any way to make my son financially responsible for *any* of the funeral costs.

I felt I had gotten the last laugh.

I explained to my son that the actions my ex's family had taken much earlier in my ex's life were now coming back to haunt them. They had caused my son hurt throughout his life because they never acknowledged him as part of their family. They had chosen that path and this was what it had led to.

When we arrived back at my son's house, as soon as he got out of the car, he hugged me and said, "I know you were awfully young when you had me, but I am glad you didn't do what a lot of mothers did during that time and give me up at birth. You gave me the father I needed in life. The person who was at the funeral home only provided the biological portion of who I am physically. You and Dad made me who I am today. I am thankful for the strong mother you have always been for me. I only wish that you had had a strong set of parents yourself through the difficult times in your life."

Those were the words I had always needed to hear. I never knew when, or if, they would ever come. I found it ironic that my ex's death provided the opportunity for my son and me to have that very conversation on the very day his DNA had been obtained.

As for my parents' non-support, that's another story.

As for my ex's funeral cost, my son was never contacted again.

As for as the DNA results, they proved who my son's biological father was, exactly as we expected. We are grateful that MS is not hereditary.

A lot was put to rest during that time.

As they say, we never know why things happen the way they do, when they do. However, eventually we figure out the reason why. It may be in an hour, the next day, or 26 years later.

CHAPTER 13

CHIAROSCURO

~ ALYESHKA HARMON ~

"Truth" is a kaleidoscope, and I embrace it in all its color and collisions. ALL of them. This piece is about living with dearly-loved adult children whose kaleidoscopes specifically exclude some of the darker colors and collisions of my own as we all come to terms with the unexpected car-crash death of their father. It is about the interplay of light and shadow, what medieval painters came to call *chiaroscuro*. The Visual Arts Encyclopedia speaks of it as "a painterly shading technique used specifically to give 2-D objects a sense of volume: that is, to make them look like three-dimensional solids ..." It is about the riddle of how to live with our respective truths, about when to keep silent in love, and when to speak in love, in those times when a three-dimensional portrait is necessary for the physical and moral health of the living.

My ex died in a December, on the threshold of Christmas. He wished to be seen as a larger-than-life figure, and in many ways, he was that person, embarking solo on excursions so extreme that few others would even contemplate undertaking them, let alone actually pulling them off. He was a gadfly conservationist. I am glad that in the last weeks of his life, he could celebrate a significant political victory won by the movement he helped to catalyze—the culmination of years of work, and one that gave hope of saving a heritage wilderness ecosystem from development. This was true and good work on his part, rightly praiseworthy.

He wrote prolifically nearly every day from mid-adolescence until the very day he died—journals, books, letters, articles for newspapers and magazines. My youngest calculated initially that there are 10,000 pages of his writing, 40 years' worth—now, with additional discoveries, it looks as if there are twice as many. He delighted in infuriating journalist friends by advising them to "just make it up" when they were uncertain about facts.

I believe the accounts of the expeditions are largely true. And I know that the public and private renditions of our domestic life never once mentioned the violence, chaos, desperation, and despair that were part of its fabric, in addition to the lyrical moments so amply chronicled.

Chiaroscuro—the interplay of brilliant light and darkest dark, "an effect of contrasted light and shadow created by light falling unevenly or from a particular direction on something..." [Google dictionary]. The thousands of pages he left behind shed an uneven light indeed, and I am trying to come to terms with that in the most wholesome, true, and loving way possible.

He wished to be seen as deeply kind—the kind of man his revered father was—and he cultivated public kindnesses. I remember sitting in the car, one of the enclosures in which our hellish moments played out, and marveling at the dexterity with which he could turn in a microsecond from cutting cruelty toward me to gracious generosity toward a neighbor. Some of the kindnesses were reminisced about at his memorial service, rightly so—but it is an incomplete portrait of the man if these are the only stories we have of him.

We had our share of hell-days when the kids were growing up, days filled with violence and shouting that I cringe to remember, and that I worry may have caused them irreparable damage. After one such day, he asked me to read his journal entry. It spoke only of sun and lake-swimming, bug-catching, and children in the late summer light. There was no mention of the savagery, no introspection about any role he may have played in its genesis, nor any role he potentially could play in preventing such scenes in the future. When I asked him about this omission, he shrugged and said simply, "It's not important."

Both during our years as a family, and also during our years of separation, my goal was to clearly point out to the kids the difference between right and wrong actions without impinging on their native deep affection for their father. I believed that affection was one of the keys to their development as full human beings, and therefore, I strove to preserve it. A flotilla of therapists, and too many wise and very patient friends, helped me to strike this balance as best I could.

In what we now know were the last months of his life, a shared building project evolved amongst him and our children. It brought peace to his soul and deepened the love in every direction. By definition, I was excluded, and I struggled, seeing that this project was setting up summers they would spend together for years to come, which would mean that I would miss out on time with the children (and also very precious playtime with grandchildren, whenever they would arrive). I struggled privately with my feelings that summer, vowing that I would NOT inflict more conflict and more angst on my children—they had seen too much already.

I am very proud that I succeeded in harnessing my reactions, and I am grateful that we do not have to live with memories of me tormenting the kids in his last months with my distress over their choice to set up what looked like future years of shared time with him that would exclude me. I am proud that I transmuted weeks of angst into a mild question to our eldest (his "adopted" non-biological son, my firstborn): since that shared project would not have come to pass if he had lived in Kansas City rather than in the remote and spectacular wilderness, and since it was a project hatched and nurtured in shared love of wilderness, what might be the shared passion that would afford me similar joyful access to him and his family? My son wrote back that he did not know in the moment, but very much appreciated the question and looked forward to discovering the answer together. I loved him for that, and I knew he was telling me the truth.

~

We spent Christmas Eve day on airplanes, converging from various far-flung points. Two of the kids had made it to the coroner's office early enough to wade through paperwork and hilarious, but macabre bureaucratic ineptitude "What do you mean you *lost* the body?", and to procure his body before the office closed. I had hunted for hours for a vehicle large enough to hold all of us, and a body, and groceries for seven for a week. We picked it up at the airport.

Eight p.m. found us wandering dazed under the Fellini-esque fluorescents of a Walmart, because it was the only possible place to get groceries at that time on Christmas Eve. The kids were cratered with grief—faces gray, the normally boisterous horseplay of reunion engulfed in silence much deeper than the mere absence of words. That, more than anything else, was my agony, for I could do nothing to lighten it. He unquestionably was the most important person in each of their lives, and in an inexplicable moment on an icy highway, he was gone forever. I could not die instead of him and I could not bring him back.

The details of the next week were the stuff of Zhivago— fittingly so, for only enormous effort could match the enormous grief. He'd always said he wanted to be laid out "to feed the animals" on the remote cabin land, so seven of us slogged into the wind through knee-deep drifts at 20 degrees below for over five miles, finally arriving at the cold dark house he'd built, to make that possible. It was a tribute rendered in seven solitudes, some bodies feverish, some deconditioned and shocked by exertion, all doggedly focused on fulfilling that wish of his.

For the purposes of this essay collection, however, the nub of it is this: we had to go through paperwork there, looking for things like bank statements and insurance documents. That meant churning through a melange of manuscripts and letters as well—anything to get a more accurate picture of his affairs. Perhaps there would even be a will. He had told the kids he intended to change it. I kept marveling at the seamless fabric of the narrative he left behind. In all those thousands of papers, there was no accurate mention of either myself or of his first partner, the mother of his first child, whom I helped to raise, and whom I consider to be one of my own, just as she and I consider each other to be sisters. There was no mention of the many ways in which we daily contributed to that mythic life in the deep wilderness, nor to his writings. It is a story in which, without mothers, life was perfect, and he was a benevolent, if beleaguered, chronicler of childhood's halcyon moments. Twining through those pages, and through his voluminous journals, was the double helix of paradisiacal renditions of childhood days at the wonderland homestead, interlaced with and spiraling around the other helix of observations that their lives would be perfect, would have been perfect, had it not been for the moms. Moms are rendered by turns as raging, erratic, mean-spirited, weak, afraid, and needy of male protection and oversight.

We have disappeared from the homestead memorabilia, we two mothers—all pictures are gone. The bonfire he made years earlier—after he realized I really would not be coming back— destroyed my clothing, the love letters I had written to him over years, the joint journal I had started with him in hopes that we could find truth by writing rather than screaming, the rough wooden spoons the kids had proudly carved for me, my baby book with its pictures of grandparents and great-grandparents, the journal I'd written to our youngest while I was pregnant with him—its ultrasound portrait showing that he unquestionably would inherit his dad's nose. Years later, I asked my ex why he burned all these things, to which he said, "Because I couldn't bear the thought that you had a life, and a life with the kids, apart from me."

My daughter-in-law was nonplused that I could walk right into the cabin, after 15 years' absence, and immediately muscle a log into the stove; perhaps nonplused as well that I am keeper of so much deep history of the place and community—and no wonder! How could she ever know I had been there at all, when I had been so perfectly erased from the place?

I had known from years of playing high-stakes child custody chess with him that he tried to undermine the kids' relationships to their mothers. But turning page after page of new and old letters to them, and of journal passages nudging them to "cut the apron strings," or to realize that their lives (and possibly their relation to him) would be vastly better if they forsook their mothers—and coming to realize how sustained an obsession this had been, over decades—was like receiving a blow to the solar plexus.

Up until this point, I had been managing to walk the *arête* of my own grief for him, and for the tragedy of his death, combined with accompanying our devastated adult children, and navigating the complex logistics of this passage. I grieved his early and unfair loss—my wish always was that he would heal, that he would learn to be kind to me, and overcome whatever monsters of the deep made it impossible for him to be kind to the women with whom he had shared home and children. Failing that, my wish was for my own life's safety and sanity.

However, turning those pages, and realizing the extent of the erasure, coupled with the distortions rendered to the children about how their childhoods had been, and who their mothers were, made me think of propaganda machines the world over, and of Hitler's observation in *Mein Kampf,* that a big lie carries "force and credibility" despite facts to the contrary in ways that a little lie never could. The "grossly impudent lie always leaves traces behind it, even after it has been nailed down ..." We, the mothers, are the facts to the contrary, the "traces" behind the lie.

Obviously, he was not a Hitler. And I do not believe that he consciously fabricated the lies—though I am not always sure about that. Rather, he wrote about life as he wished it to be—over and over and over again. At one point, I turned to our eldest as we were reading and said, "This is hard for me." When he tossed his head and rolled his eyes, I realized that it was not the time and place for me to come to terms with the new awareness of how single-mindedly my ex had worked to undermine the kids' relationships with me and with his first partner, nor would the children probably ever be able to discuss it. Their own needs for the superhero dad, variously refracted, would preclude any ability to tolerate a much more complex portrait of the man. It was already an abundance of graciousness on their parts that not one of them ever made it seem strange that I was here with them, deep in this time, in the home from which I'd been barred by the man with whom I ultimately broke communication, in sadness, and as the only measure I knew that would preserve sanity for all of us.

His blind spot was living intimacy with the women who bore his children—and that same blind spot, it was whispered at his service, came to threaten his conservation work as well because it extended to the women who supported his work and collaborated with him.

Our children's adulation of him, combined with the howling mistral of grief, the return to the home I'd cherished, and the life I'd helped to create for over a decade, and the eerily perfect life depicted in the journals, made me doubt my sanity at times during those dark, still, frigid days. Now, if I start to question my sanity, a circle of friends, both men and women, remember him with a flaming anger I no longer feel, because I feel first the kids' grief, and my own helpless yearning to heal it. Friends held, and continue to hold, the other pieces of memory and kaleidoscope that the kids cannot—many with a fury that has long since played out in me.

Yet, and yet—in those first days, I longed for a Speaker for the Dead[1]—one who could give full account of the deceased, showing with compassion and clarity how the roots of his

---

1   Speaker for the Dead is the name of a novel by Orson Scott Card. He describes the function of such a Speaker, which is to delve deeply into the life of the one who has died, and to tell the story of that life in fullness, so that the compassion that inevitably comes with knowing the entire story of any one person's journey can emerge.

worst moments lay in his own grievous childhood wounding, and how these deserve our compassion no less than our awareness. Who of us wouldn't want and need that? Where was the person who could speak the comprehensive truth of this life, its goodness, badness, and contradictions? Who could bring dimension and fullness to the 2-D superhero cartoon?

And, with regard to the children, why would it even matter?

Partly, it matters because familial lies or secrets can germinate underground and surface as unhappy patterns in the lives of another generation. If the superhero's clay feet are never spoken of, then how can children and grandchildren ever know when they are living out an earlier template? How can they ever know that they are free not to repeat the mistakes of their forebears, free to make different choices? When does that larger-than-life myth about who he was become the tyrannical standard that they can never hope to equal?

I am publishing pseudonymously, though my children are aware that I am writing this piece. When does my mercy in not pushing them to admit the missing bits of the kaleidoscope become collusion with the lie? I will wrestle with this question for a long time to come.

In honesty, I have to say that it matters to me as a woman that our contributions to our cultural superheroes' endeavors be known. My ex's deeds were extraordinary, and they were under-written much of the way by myself and by his first partner—in later years, by the children as well, and in public life, by several women who kindly and skillfully modulated his rough edges. I use the plural—"superheroes"—here because I want this essay to include OUR—women's—contributions to the many superheroes worshiped by our culture; my story is not unique. The collective story begins with feeding him and bedding him, sometimes earning the money by which he is fed and bedded, often by tending to the daily details that relentlessly eat up hours as well as spaciousness of thought. It continues in our deep listening, the midwifery by which his deepest thoughts and most cherished dreams emerge. Virginia Woolf spoke of this as a mirroring function:

> Women have served all these centuries as look-ing-glasses possessing the magic and delicious power of reflecting the figure of man at twice its natural size ... Whatever may be their use in civilised [sic] societies, mirrors are essential to all violent and heroic action. That is why Napoleon and Mussolini both insist so emphatically upon the inferiority of women, for if they were not inferior, they would cease to enlarge. That serves to explain in part the necessity that women so often are to men... And it serves to explain how restless they are under [a woman's] criticism;... For if she begins to tell the truth, the figure in the looking-glass shrinks; his fitness in life is diminished. How is he to go on ... unless he can see himself at breakfast and at dinner at least twice the size he really is?[2]

~

It also matters to me that my ex, like many other environmentalists, could truly commune with Mother Earth and champion her protection, yet in his worst moments, he could virtually clear-cut the mothers of his children.

---

2   Virginia Woolf, 1929. *A Room of One's Own*. Harcourt Brace Jovanovich.

If, as Jung said, the shadow is "the invisible saurian tail that man still drags behind him," which, "carefully amputated . . . becomes the healing serpent of the mysteries," then I want us to see both darkness and light with kaleidoscopic complexity and humility.[3] I want us to live in Jung's "House of the Gatherings," the place inhabited by "someone brave enough to withdraw all his projections ... someone conscious of a pretty thick shadow ..." Such a person, wrote Jung, can no longer locate problems exclusively "out there," but must gather them in and confront them as complex fictions manufactured by a self-hell—bent on protection from awareness of its own evil.

I agree with Jung that those who dwell in that House of Gatherings have "done something real for the world ... [have] succeeded in shouldering at least an infinitesimal part of the gigantic, unsolved social problems of our day."[4] But there is more to it. The shadow-reptilian tail is helped to become "the healing serpent of the mysteries" when not only the cultural superheroes but also those around them change the looking-glass by telling a fuller version of the truth. Virginia Woolf again:

> For if she begins to tell the truth, the figure in the looking-glass shrinks ... The looking-glass vision is of supreme importance because it charges the vitality; it stimulates the nervous system. Take it away and man may die, like the drug fiend deprived of his cocaine.

3   Carl Jung, *The Integration of the Personality*, 1939.
4   Carl Jung, "Psychology and Religion. In Collected Works 11: *Psychology and Religion: West and East*, 1938, p.140).

If we end the silence about the Great Man's cruelty to his wife (and also the silence about her contributions), if we learn that many, perhaps most, of the champions of the earth—no less than the transcendent artists and apostles of non-violence—caused great pain to their wives[5], perhaps the looking-glass figure shrinks, but then don't we also perhaps learn something essential about human nature (or at least about patriarchal society)? And could the mirror that is "essential to violent and heroic actions" become a different mirror, perhaps one that enlarges wholeness, sanity, and what it takes for everyone to flourish?

Silence about a woman's support of a Great Man's Great Work is intimately tied into silence about the Great Man's cruelty to her—in both cases, the reality of her life is invisible.[6] Woolf will again help us to see why this matters, as she muses on what would have happened if Shakespeare had had a sister. That sister would have been unseen, and suppressed, and at times abused. She would have died anonymously. But—and this is the crucial point—this woman, this sister,

> ... *still lives. She lives in you and in me, and in many other women who are not here tonight, for they are washing up the dishes and putting the children to bed. But she lives; for great poets do not die; they are continuing presences; they need only the opportunity to walk among us in the flesh. This opportunity, as I think, it is now coming within your power to give her.*

5   See for examples *Bearing the Cross: Martin Luther King Jr. and the Southern Christian Leadership Conference* by David Garrow (William Morrow Paperbacks 2004) and *Gandhi's Truth* by Erik Erikson (W. W. Norton 1969).

6   These issues also hold for persons of color in white culture, for they also are the diminished other that makes the Great Man appear larger.

Think on that! WE have the power to bring her to life, that brilliant woman who died in despair! Woolf states,

> *For my belief is that if ... we have the habit of freedom and the courage to write exactly what we think; if we ... see human beings ... in relation to reality ... then the opportunity will come and the dead poet who was Shakespeare's sister will put on the body which she has so often laid down. Drawing her life from the lives of the unknown who were her fore-runners ... she will be born. As for her coming without that preparation, without that effort on our part, without that determination that when she is born again, she shall find it possible to live and write her poetry, that we cannot expect, for that would be impossible. But I maintain that she would come if we worked for her.*

So the work that we do, by un-silencing our truths—spoken, written and sung—forges a new mirror. It creates the culture in which "Judith Shakespeare," that imagined/real/composite woman who is each one of us, can live and create.

Books like this one, books that give voice to what has been silent, and that make kaleidoscopes of women's truths, help to create that culture. That hope moves me beyond my native reserve, to write as honestly as I can, even though veiled by the pseudonym my children have requested.

~

The National Center for Health Statistics tells us that half of U.S. marriages end in divorce. Furthermore, we do not know how many of the still-married are barely hanging on.

The Hallmark-card version of marriage leaves out at least half the story, so in an aging society, there are many of us who have or will confront being "the ex" within the community of mourning and remembrance. It is a complicated role. We also will participate in memorials at which ex-spouses or ex-partners are present. Briefly, here are some things I have learned, practical things to do if you are part of the after-death gatherings and an ex is included:

- Be aware that he or she loved that person once, possibly as much as you have, and that he or she is present now because of that original love, however complicated it became over time.

- Please make room for the ex, and meet his or her eyes in kindness.

- Please realize that his or her grief is real, and that your knowledge of what really happened between the one who died and the one still living is extremely limited.

- Please acknowledge the ex as someone who also was important in the life we now memorialize, in ways that you will never know.

I was fortunate enough to experience all of these things from family and community, despite my fears that I would not. I feared that as carrier of the shadow-story, I would not be welcome—but I was, and it was unexpected grace for which I am forever grateful.

~

In sorrow, we laid him out, as he wished. I gasped when I saw the sculpted beauty of his dead body, and watched in surprise as the old longing and welcome surged forward in my own. Gladly would I have lain down in the snow to take him tenderly into my arms.

Our physicality—the meals, the wilderness surroundings and the demands it made on us, the love-making—healed me from a disease I had been told was life-threatening. His fear that if I got well, I would leave, made him controlling and violent. I used to tell him, only partly teasing, that if we could just put duct tape over our mouths, we would be able to live in peace.

The relationship healed me, and it stole my soul. It was a dreadful *chiaroscuro* riddle, the white-hot coal stuck in the throat that I could neither swallow down nor cough up. I stayed because I wanted to repay him for the gift of health restored, and I stayed because I didn't want the children to undergo the pyrotechnics that a divorce undoubtedly would (and did) bring. I stayed because I loved him. I stayed, hoping things would get better. I left when I finally realized that, one way or another, this was going to cost the children a mother, and I did not agree that their lives would get better if I died.

And now with his unexpected death and the revelations left behind in his writings, the riddle returned and re-configured: how to support the adult children's needs for his simple goodness as they grieve, while holding space for my own more complicated truth and grief?

~

I have a scrap of clothing that he was wearing when he died; it was bloody and so I hid it from the children. I could not bear to throw it out, nor could I bear to wash out his blood and let it run down the drain, or throw the bloody water out onto the frozen snow. There will be a moment at some later time, and a white-hot fire, and I will release the cloth and his blood to the transmutation of the elements. But for now, I hold them in secret, still clinging to the vibrational token of our most intimate sharing.

~

Months later, we returned to see what had become of him. All that remained was one drop of blood, a hair or two, and a single wolf-print fading in the spring snow. I believe he would be pleased now to be a wolf freely traversing vast areas of wilderness. It pleases me to think that perhaps a she-wolf took him, a mother—and perhaps he gave her the means to nurse her young in the sparse late winter, sustenance he could rarely give to the mothers of his own children.

~

I watch the wolves now. My inbox has become flooded with updates from the wolf conservationists. I pay heed to their news, signing petitions and donating when I can. A new fierce protectiveness of the wolf-tribe sings in my veins—that is another truth-piece for the kaleidoscope. Let them live! Do not kill them! Mysteriously, unbidden, they are our riddles. They are both light and shadow, as are we. Wandering far and wild, they both endanger our lambs and imprint wholeness into the very earth[7]—they are his kin, and they are ours.

---

7   Please visit https://www.youtube.com/watch?v=ysa5OBhXz-Q (*How Wolves Change Rivers*) to see how literally true this statement is.

Chapter 14

Loves Lives On

~ Rima Star ~

I first met Jerry in 1980. He was a husband, father, and business executive who made an impression on me when I was visiting other family members at his home. He was a tall hulk of a man who seemed to dwell primarily in one section of the house—what we, as a culture, would later come to call a "man cave." When he walked through the larger house, where many of us were having our own conversations, he kept his focus forward and down, as if bringing his "man cave" with him. No one attempted to cross his path.

In 1985, I received a phone call in which he said he had just read a chapter I wrote in someone's book about my experiences with a technique called rebirthing. He said he was ready to do the ten-session process and reminded me that I had been in his home those years earlier. Would I work with him? I had to think about it—my second baby was about nine months old at the time, and I had not gone fully back to my consultation work. Eventually, after an interview, we worked out a plan and began the session experience. Through this work, I help people look at their early life (conception-bonding) for experiences that turn into imprinted "messages" that underlie and may inform a person's present-time life.

I remember Jerry shared from his sessions with me that he felt "filled with the spirit of breath." He said, "I can imagine when it is time to pass into the next world, I can have 'a seamless breath' from this life into the next." I could feel how much that meant to him, and how real the feeling of peace was for him. He completed the ten sessions and our lives went on with a greater appreciation and knowledge of each other.

A few years later, he called and invited me to participate in a prosperity and business success group he was starting. I knew some of the other people in the group. I thought about it, asked family and friends for their opinions, and decided that as a busy therapist, wife, and mother of two, it would be beneficial for me to take time to be in a group for my own purposes. The group met twice a month, discussing topics and sharing experiences regarding our relationship to prosperity, spirituality, and business success. We all became better friends. Jerry—"the bear" as he often referred to himself—became a more and more significant figure in my life.

The holistic education group that my husband, Steven, and I had begun in the early 1980s had eight key teachers who gave seminars all over the United States and a few other countries. But over time, what had started out as a beneficial group informing others about holistic options for health and wellness, slowly became skewed in a direction that I would describe now as "ungrounded spiritual sensationalism." I later realized that this was part of a phenomenon of awakening to direct spiritual experience throughout the United States. I see it now as akin to learning to walk, or handle a great deal more "spiritual energy" than a person had access to before—not always coherent, steady, or kind. Over the years, as I felt more and more in the minority within the group leadership, I began to integrate the changes I was seeing into a new reality for myself. I was grateful to be connected with my new prosperity group, whose members gave me a chance to gain perspective on what I was experiencing.

My business and personal world slowly eroded into something I did not feel in alignment with, or as a beneficial environment in which to raise my children. During this time, my connection with my "independent" friends grew, and Jerry became a significant listener as I made some of the hard decisions I was facing. In 1987, as I pulled further and further away from my former colleagues, "the group" as I came to call them did their best (or worst!) to keep me and my financial support involved. I thought that surely Steven, father of our now three children, would follow us when I bravely announced to him that I wanted us to leave our connection with the group and work independently. To my surprise (at the time), he would not leave and blamed me for choosing a path he saw as inferior.

The process of dissolving a ten-year marriage was fraught with feelings of fear and angst. Underneath the fear, I managed to be a warrior and champion of what I knew in my heart as the best choice for our family. I became a "Mama bear," defending the well-being of my children and discovered strengths I didn't know I had. Jerry, as one of my trusted independent friends, grew as a stabilizing point in this process, encouraging and supportive of the choices I was making.

As this period of dissolution and divorce finalized, I was able to breathe easier and look at my life from a new place of hope. It was during this time that Jerry's and my relationship grew from friendship into more—a possibility for a new start for all of us.

From a poem he wrote me at the time:

There is within every person
A voice that speaks

With absolute purity and innocence
Of universal truth.
We are, each divine one of us a medium for this
essential
Intrinsic good that resides
At our core
Thus, we speak without condition
And by Grace
The harmony of innocence
Nourishing all beings.

Eventually, I was independent again.

Jerry made three glorious marriage proposals to me in three beautiful locations, feeling that the number three was spiritually significant. I said yes each time. We married in July 1989, in a home ceremony of our creation. His son, Rob, and daughter, Kei, and my three children, Mela, Orien, and Hank were witnesses. A community of close family and friends celebrated with music, readings, poetry, and great food on a beautiful sunny July 1 day. A dear friend of ours, who was a retired Episcopal priest, officiated. I truly believe we had the best intentions. Jerry took, or added, the name Jeremiah as part of our ceremony because he felt that it represented his connection to his spiritual self.

In the previous years of the 1980s, I had experienced the births of my three children, and the deaths of both of my parents, at the early ages of 62 for my dad, and 64 for my mom—and a divorce from Steven. My mom died one week before the birth of my second daughter in 1984. Those experiences were the catalyst for telling my story in *The Healing Power of Birth* (1986).

Jerry's 1980s included highs and lows as an owner and executive of an insurance company, and the dissolution and divorce of his first 20+ years of marriage, and the changes that made for all of them, including his two wonderful adult children. He was attracted during these years to the study of various forms of meditation centered on mystical Christianity, "personal growth" philosophies, and bringing that type of consciousness into the business world. He created a newsletter that went to recipients of insurance from his company to 30,000 or more people entitled, *I Choose Health*. He also was exploring the practice of macrobiotics and other approaches to health and food. Community gatherings, including dance, were integral parts of our life together.

He had nicknames for each of my children, which they love to this day. They called him "Jer-Bear." Many weekends, there were gatherings around and in the pool—Jerry as "the whale," and my children and most everyone else as "the dolphins." These days were followed by large community-created meals that reminded me of the extended family gatherings I had enjoyed as a child growing up in Texas.

During this time (and for 20 years) in my role as teacher/therapist, I offered a healing experience in the Florida Keys centered on the theme "Living in the Heart of the Wave." It included personal processing and play in the open ocean, which we called the "dolphins' playground." One summer, Jerry and I, with my children, staying a week longer for family time, had an especially meaningful experience.

One of the members of our group was walking on the beach by our house at dawn. She saw a small whale beached in the shallow water, while swimming further out and going in a semi-circle was a baby whale making crying sounds. Apparently, the baby whale could not get into the shallow, or was hesitant to do so. We later found out that they were sperm whales. Our friend ran back to the house and told us to come and help. Jer-Bear, my children Mela, Orien, Hank and I gathered a few things and headed over.

We were some of the first people there. The call went out to Marine Mammal Rescue, and more and more people began to arrive. Most attention seemed centered on the mother. Jerry, being whale-like himself at 6'7", was eagerly invited to come into the water and help so the mother could stay above water and breathe until Marine Rescue arrived. My children were pulling on his arms and leading him to the ocean saying, "Jer-Bear, help the whale!" It was a beautiful sight with the sun coming up, the sand sparkling, and three relatively small, excited, determined children hanging and pulling on this whale of a man to help the mother whale.

I was doing my best to entrain my intentions with the baby whale, and let her or him know that his mother was being helped. Then my kids came back with someone who seemed to be "in the know" and I said, "What about the baby?" That resulted in the baby being reached and scooped up and brought to us. He/she was put in an inflatable boat under a palm tree (which provided some shade) and the Star family became the baby's caregivers for the day. Jerry would take breaks from holding the mother whale and come join us for food, water, and a little rest.

The kids and I started talking to the baby, and I suggested that the children, with their minds, send the baby pictures of the mom being helped and also letting the mom know her baby was safe. We laid our hands on the baby. One of my children suggested we sing (of course!). I think we started with some Hindu chants and then got into nursery rhymes. Others would stop and join in for a while. I was stroking the baby's face, children chanting, and suddenly, the baby cried and his tears were flowing over my hand. I was amazed and deeply touched. So were my children. I hadn't known that whales cried real tears.

The baby stuck out his tongue, wrapped it around my finger and started suckling. I cried and my children said, "Mom, he's going to be okay now." It was almost sunset when both mother and baby were safely in the rescue truck and taken to the marine mammal sanctuary to heal and recover and eventually return to the ocean. We had taken turns napping in the shade, going for food and water, helping other people, and of course, being caregivers—doulas—for the baby whale. The five of us walked home in the sunset feeling like participants in the circle of life.

These two years were an oasis in the midst of all that had happened in both of our lives during that decade, and all that was about to happen, especially for Jerry. It seemed that I had been through my "trial of fire," and he was entering into his.

His journey centered on his professional life and business. The details have faded into the past and don't require searching for at this time. I remember that they involved disagreements with partners, loss of business, being on the news, lawsuits that stretched on for years, and most likely many other troubling things unknown to me.

As each week and month passed, he withdrew further and further from interaction with just about everybody, including me. He also, one by one, let go of things he had enjoyed doing—

cooking, dancing, writing, gardening, and visiting friends. Habits of meditation and reading books on spirituality and mysticism also fell by the wayside. I was a witness and as much support as I could be, while running a household, maintaining a private practice, writing, and of course, most importantly, being a mom.

Behaviors that did surface—drinking, smoking, brooding, isolating—showed me sides of Jerry I had not known existed. One day, after my children came home from school, one of them said, "Mom, should I go take Jerry his drink (i.e., alcoholic beverage)?" I was startled and said, "No, that's not necessary." Abruptly, I woke up to the unspoken effects of the changing home environment on my children. I was committed to providing an environment where unhealthy substances and behaviors were not a part of their daily lives.

After a passionate plea and attempted discussion with Jerry that evening, I proclaimed that I and my children would move into another house in their old neighborhood. When he was in that home, different rules would apply. I said I would be with him in his home, but not with the kids, until things were different. I was actually blown away by my strength and determination in making that statement and following through within days.

Several years passed with us living in this two-home system. The adjustment after I made the proclamation and followed through was a journey filled with challenges and new levels of grief for me—and gradual acceptance that I needed to let go completely from seeing Jerry. On New Year's Eve of 1999, I made the decision and let him know I was going into the new decade without spending time with him. I did. I placed my focus on being the best parent I could be for my now-teenage children.

He was not happy with my decision, and continued to check in with me. Very slowly, his check-ins slowed to only once or twice a year. He did keep in communication with the children, taking them out for birthdays and other events.

In 2007, my children and longtime women's group friends planned a surprise birthday party at my friend Robbie's home for my 60th birthday celebration—the start of a new decade of my life. There were many people present. Part of the process was a ritual that Robbie had creatively designed for me.[1] It took place outdoors, where I was met by my children or my friends at separate stations around Robbie's large, circular driveway. Each station represented a decade of my life. I was asked to report on the highlights of each decade and what I had learned during that period. As I spoke, often people would call out, "Don't forget this or that." When I received approval from the group via a lot of clapping, I moved on to the next decade station.

At about the third station, I noticed that Jerry was in the crowd. He towered over everyone else and was rather hard to miss. Hmmm ... What was the conspiracy that got him invited? I wondered.

When I came to the stations for the decades of the 1980s and 1990s, I was worried about what my friends would require me to report before they would let me pass on. If it were in this day and age, I might have been texting, "OMG—help me!" I do

---

1   See *How To Create and Perform an Effective Stage 4 Ritual: Things to Remember and Include,* the Appendix to *The Power of Ritual* by Robbie Davis-Floyd Charles D. Laughlin, 2016.

not remember what I said. I do remember that I summoned all of the equanimity and goodwill I could muster to mention some highlights relative to Jerry, and completely lost them right after I said them. I remember that Jerry seemed quite relieved and friendly. I most likely spoke with him during the party, but don't recall. I decided not to be mad at anyone for him being there, but to accept that perhaps it was time to face his significance in my life.

Since his business losses in the 1990s, Jerry had re-created himself as a farmer with 90 acres devoted to organic egg production and a growing organic feed mill. To this day, his mill supplies organic farmers throughout the region. His egg cartons say, "Laid by happy hens living in organic pastures." Now, his son and family continue the business and the traditions he started there.

Jerry consistently invited me to come visit. The kids would go occasionally, but I hadn't been out there in years. He also started stopping by my home after that birthday event, and we began to chat again. One time, at a Christmas visit in 2009, with my children, I remember thinking, "Okay, Rima, maybe it's a good idea to review yourself in relation to Jerry to see how far you have come in your healing."

There is a quote from the ever-popular Anonymous: "Holding resentment is like eating poison and then waiting for the other person to keel over" (you can find it in Alan Cohen's book *A Deep Breath of Life*). My inner muse says, "Sometimes, our resentment drives us to safety, then there comes a moment when it's time to get out of the car." I thought that perhaps this was that moment for me.

Jerry loved to be the master of the kitchen and whip up farm fresh meals (as opposed to cooking together). I started going out to the farm for dinner every so often. He told me how hurt he had been that I did not respond when he first faced the news of his cancer diagnosis. He later was in remission for a number of years and then it resurfaced. I listened to his story and sharing of his feelings and journey—a path that led him to some amazing people and experiences. It was good to learn about the people who loved him and participated with him in this journey, and all the places it led him. I would add my "healing juju," as he called it, by having a special altar for him at my home and adding my support to the mix.

I did my best in those visits to review and face the various types of unforgiveness I still found within myself. I would joke with myself and close friends that this was my "therapy" time. Truly, it gave me plenty to face within myself, and became a deeply healing experience for me (and still is).

We had some ongoing fun watching and commenting on the *Dancing with the Stars* television show. I would go out to his farm about once a month so we could watch the show together. We would also watch old movies that we both loved. And of course, we would comment on the state of our children—his two, their spouses, and his grandchildren, and my three, whom I was calling "adult children" to help myself get used to that concept. Jerry and I were very grateful when my daughter, Orien, met the man she knew she would marry—Andy—and they both were able to spend an afternoon at the farm in October 2012. (Orien and Andy married in 2014.)

Jerry was very pleased, and rightfully so, about the creation of the farm and egg and feed business. He said he wanted to be a contributor to the betterment of people and the planet. In the past, he would refer to himself as a "sheep in wolf's clothing," and was writing a book about being a mystic in business. I think he was attempting to come full circle from his earlier perceptions of himself, and be about the business of contribution. I reminded him of a vision I had of him early on in our marriage—I saw him living on the land with his hands in the dirt, and doing something artistic, like sculpting. At the time, he thought that was ridiculous. When we reconnected, I had to claim a few points for that vision, since he had found peace and creative satisfaction on the farm. He agreed. We had to laugh that he had gone from a suit-wearing business executive to an overall-wearing farmer, and I had gone from being a healer-helper-breath teacher to a business executive providing oxygen-infused products to the marketplace.

He had been cancer-free for a number of years. Toward the end of 2012, he was once again diagnosed with cancer. He said he was done with medical treatments—and so began his journey of acceptance of transitioning into spirit. As with most things with Jerry/Jeremiah, he was in charge and had a plan. People lined up to take him where he needed to go and prepare his home in the ways he wanted it to be. He decided he wanted a "green" burial on his farm, and began to bring together his ideas for his post-death Celebration of Life. I'm sure this news radiated out into many communities of people touched by Jerry.

I see in my journal that I spent time with him on the morning of July 6, 2013. He completed his transition on August 6, the month before his 77th birthday. That July day, I brought him red roses, coral flowers in a red vase, and a book of Hafiz poetry. He had on black shorts, a cinnamon/coral shirt, red sheets on the bed, and the walls still painted a bright, strong blue—as was the blouse I was wearing.

The organic garden nearby was in full bloom, the sun streaming through the windows. I thought what a colorful, vibrant scene this was for a man who truly loved the physicality of being human. Opposite to his bed was a table piled high with books he loved—notably anything by Thomas Merton, and other gifts people had brought him, pictures of his Mom, Dad, brother (all of whom had already passed into spirit), and his children and grandchildren.

I asked him what he wanted and he said a cup of tea. I brought it to him and we talked. He told me he really wanted to see Mela, Orien, and Hank, if at all possible, and I said I would let them know. We talked about the beautiful day we all had together in October when he met Andy, Orien's fiancé. He told me how glad he was that I had stopped refusing to see him. I laughed and said, "Proof that miracles do exist."

He asked, "Would you give me a massage and lay your healing hands on me?" I said yes, prepared the space with his favorite oils, and ended by holding him in my arms while he slept. Because of his height, and also our whale rescue experience, I would call him my "whale man." That's how I felt about him on this day—holding him while he slept peacefully.

Someone from hospice was coming on Monday mornings to check in with him. I agreed to be there for the next two Mondays by 8 a.m., when she arrived. Mela came with me the next Monday, and Hank the following Monday. Each had their special farewell time with Jerry. Orien was scheduled to arrive July 28.

The next two Mondays, I met with the hospice person, who was usually somewhat frustrated with Jerry not exactly being receptive to her suggestions. Then I would meet with Rob and

Amy when they arrived a little later. We would discuss what the hospice nurse said would be helpful and how to convince Jerry to agree. One example—having a walker near the bed, and then, near the end, a wheelchair available in the room. Jerry was managing his visitor schedule via texting, and could still bring forth the "growling bear" part of his personality when he wanted to.

Rob, Amy, and their boys started staying at the farm. His daughter, Kei, and her mom, Jerry's first wife, Karen, arrived from California. By the time Orien arrived on July 28, it was debatable whether she should/could go out there. I told her that if Jerry wasn't answering texts anymore, that was a signal that it might be beyond the time for a visit. I told her I would call and ask, but she said she felt comfortable with the memory of seeing him that October day. She said she knows Jerry loves her, and she loves him.

Rob and Amy sent out regular updates those last couple of weeks, with pictures of all of them sitting around the dining table. I was grateful that their core Cunningham family had ten or more days together, and could spend special moments with their dad, holding him, and helping him in his transition.

Many of us, his community of friends, were "holding space" for him wherever we were.

Jerry/Jeremiah made his transition on August 6, 2013.

True to form, he had planned his Celebration of Life, including a four-color program, and the people who would conduct the celebration and provide readings, poetry, and song. It was held on his farm in the beautiful morning sun, a tent set up near where he would have his green burial by a beautiful old tree on an island of grass in the circular driveway leading up to the house. He asked that a granite bench eventually be constructed there, with selected quotes from Thomas Merton to be inscribed.

Orien flew in from Colorado. The four of us—Mela, Orien, Hank, and I—headed out to the farm the day of the celebration. We arrived early so we could connect with his family, and because there was a viewing in the house, as he had asked, for those who chose to see his body one last time.

I had been there the day before, and was able to visit with Karen, his first wife, who came in from California with Kei. I see her as a wise woman and friend. It was comforting for me to be with her (and I believe she felt the same). I felt like we knew without speaking how much we share, and how truly we both wanted to be there for our respective children. I was equally happy to visit with Kei (her wonderful brood of eight children were in California with their dad). I felt proud of her as the person and parent she had become. I felt the same toward Rob and Amy and their boys, Finn and Barton. They all expressed happiness at seeing our Star family and catching up with Mela, Orien, and Hank.

I remember when people were going over to the area where the tent was set up and there were chairs, my inner voice was saying, "Oh, I want my family to be included." We were standing in the circle of people around the tent. The next thing I knew, Rob was coming over and saying, "Rima, why don't you and the kids sit here?" So there we were—Family Number One in the front row, Family Number Two behind them, and his most recent special partner graciously and beautifully conducting the celebration. I had to think, "Jerry/Jeremiah, you big bear and whale of a man—you have done something really right! Rest in peace."

The party, food, visiting, and stories that followed would certainly have made his heart happy. It was a blessing to have people come up to me and my children, and share memories from the time they knew my children as little ones. Several people from our circle of friends in the past made a point to tell Hank, Mela, and Orien that they knew that Jerry loved them with all his heart. Those words and actions and acknowledgements were medicine for me and for them. So many times, I had felt pushed out and powerless to have any assistance I offered received during those very trying years. I believe the gathering, as rightfully so for a Celebration of Life, was healing for all. My children were beaming and loved hearing stories and sharing memories. They told me that they never doubted that Jerry loved them—more heart medicine for me.

Here are selections from the two pages Jerry wrote about facing this transition:

> *One of my favorite things to do was prepare for an important trip.*
>
> *Now I have the privilege to be conscious, to prepare for the ultimate trip, a transition into another reality—another way of being.*
>
> *All the others that I prepared for included my ego,*
>
> *And all its insatiable needs.*
>
> *Now I seem to breathe a different breath when imagining my new trip.*

Later he says,

But the main gift for me in my End of Life Transition,

Is to just imagine, with an open heart and unburdened mind,

What my new eyes will see as my consciousness continues in another world.

I imagine it will be like holding hands with my friends or my children, Feeling really loved and OK—

Now as I look back at that experience of a year and a half ago, I see the healing in my life, and believe that is true within both our families. My children and I have connected with and interacted with Rob and Amy, and dear friends who are involved with the farm, and friends from the past. We attended the Thanksgiving Day tradition held at the farm. We all felt included. I sat for a while on the beautiful Texas granite bench with its inscriptions, looking at the farmhouse and land beyond, and very much felt his presence. Now I have the sneaking suspicion that feeling may be a mirror image of the deep and abiding presence of love always within and available to me. For all these things, I am grateful.

Jeremiah, I see you sustained by the unbounded and seamless breath of love.

References

Davis-Floyd, R., & Laughlin, C.D. (2016). *The power of ritual.* Daily Grail Press.

Star, R. (1986). *The healing power of birth.* Star Publishing. Available through RimaStar.com or on Amazon.

CHAPTER 15

CONCLUSION:
THE END IS JUST THE BEGINNING

The ex-husbands whose ex-wives write about their deaths in this book died from multiple causes, including suicide, murder, drug abuse, mental illness, brain damage, a heart attack, and a car crash. Life happens. Death happens. It's hard to write a conclusion to this book because, in many ways, it is just the beginning of the story. The beginning of the silence being broken. The beginning of women stepping out and admitting to the hurt and anger and grief they feel when an ex-spouse dies.

Whether you had children with your ex or not, you shared some of the most intimate moments imaginable—moments that others will never know. Now, after the funerals or memorials, and perhaps in the midst of raising children who lost their father, you are left to question why. Why do I feel the way I do? Why am I angry? Why do I not get that last final chance to reconcile the hurt between us? And why am I left out of the family, when I was such a huge part of their lives?

From Robyn's chapters in Part I, we learn about the intense suffering an ex-wife can undergo in the extraordinarily difficult circumstance of her ex-husband's suicide—the self-blame that can beset us, the horrible responsibility of being the one to have to tell your child that his father has died, and the ongoing years of struggle to help your child deal with his father's death, and also to help yourself work through the blame, shame, and guilt—if you hadn't left him, would he still be alive? The peace that Robyn and her son eventually found, and the ways in which they found that peace, can serve our readers as a guiding light.

From Robbie's chapter at the beginning of Part 2, we learn how hard it can be for an ex-wife to find any space and place to be part of a family process of grieving—especially because she had actually believed/imagined that she was a full part of that family. Her chapter recounts her hurt and confusion over being left out of all plans and family involvement, and her struggle to find her space and place for appropriate grieving within the elusive "family" context. She concludes with a brief description of her lengthy efforts to replace the anger she felt toward her ex for oh-so-many things, as well as toward herself for the mistakes she had made in the marriage, into an eventually successful "quest for forgiveness."

Kirsten Dehner's chapter speaks about re-discovering her ex-husband's presence in old artifacts that not only illuminate her home, but also call up long-suppressed memories of childhood wounds that had crippled her marriage, unexpectedly transformed through the act of writing and imagination. Annette Birchard teaches much about the ongoing effects of bitterness and rage, how very hard it is to let go and find peace, and how to keep on living when that kind of enlightenment is simply not within our reach. Like Annette's and Robbie's exes, Aleyska Harmon's ex-husband had his dark, "Dr. Jekyll" side and like them, Aleyshka had to do the hard work of dealing with her own confusion, rage, and pain without inflicting all those emotions on the children involved.

We are not saints, Dear Readers. Sometimes anger and bitterness are all we have left, yet we know we must struggle to let go and forgive, because if we continue to internalize that anger and bitterness, it may well come back to bite us in ways that can disable us profoundly and leave us unable to find peace and happiness again.

Like so many women, Aleyskha also has to struggle with the negative legacies left by her ex to his sons—might they become the abusers their father showed them how to be? She asks, "When does my mercy in not pushing them to admit the missing bits of the kaleidoscope become collusion with the lie?" answering, "I will wrestle with this question for a long time to come."

The chapters by Carol Wheeler, Laurie Wimmer, and Rima Star compellingly reveal how much we can still love our exes, no matter who they become nor how they behave. There are so many reasons for divorce—sometimes you divorce because you no longer love each other, and sometimes you divorce for other reasons, yet find that the love is ongoing—sometimes to your surprise, as Rima did. Her chapter recounts her experiences of reconnecting as friends with her ex many years after their divorce, and the sweetness that permeated their lives and those of their respective families as a result. Like Carol, Laurie, and Rima, Robbie found that her love for her ex was ongoing. Yet, as we ex-wives know, love is often not enough to sustain a marriage. In this era, when divorce is so common, we come to realize that there has to be more to a marriage than love. Shared interests, shared friends, and above all, mutual support for one another's careers, desires, and dreams are crucial to a sustainable marriage. Amazingly, most of our chapter authors found all of that in future mates—there is always hope!

From Melanie's chapter, we learn that you and your children can suffer from an "ex" who never actually married you, nor was your partner in any sense. Melanie calls him her "ex" as a shorthand, explaining that he was only the "baby daddy" whose sperm resulted in the birth of their son—a son who neither he nor his family wanted. Yet, he in death came massively into their lives when the funeral home expected their son to pay for the funeral costs for a father whom he had never met! Given the new reproductive technologies, which enable people to have children via eggs and sperm from others and surrogates to carry and birth the fetus, we can expect many more such complications in the future.

The importance of being included in the funeral or Memorial Celebration is a recurrent theme throughout the contributions. It was at her ex's Memorial that Robbie finally found her space and her place in the welcoming embraces of old and dear friends; Robyn, Annette, Alyeshka, and Rima experienced much the same. In contrast, to her ongoing pain and hurt, Laurie and her son were excluded from her ex's service, as were many of his friends and supporters, so she ended up organizing one of her own. It did help her to heal, but also created another sharp hurt when key family members chose not to attend the celebration she held. To those attending post-death gatherings of any sort in which an ex *is* included, in her chapter Alyeshka offered some excellent advice that we think important to repeat here:

- Be aware that he or she loved that person once, possibly as much as you have, and that he or she is present now because of that original love, however complicated it became over time.

- Please make room for the ex, and meet his or her eyes in kindness.

- Please realize that his or her grief is real, and that your knowledge of what really happened between the one who died and the one still living is extremely limited.

- Please acknowledge the ex as someone who also was important in the life we now memorialize, in ways that you will never know.

To those ends, we return to the last sentence of the eloquent quote from Laurie's chapter that we included in the Introduction: *If the circle of love is honored, it should be wide enough to include all who loved and were loved.*

This book is just a start, but we believe it is a good one. We hope this book can change the way we think about grief and ex-spouses for the better. Maybe it will only impact a few people, but maybe, just maybe it will start to create a larger perspective on blended families. Maybe it will help us to heal our hearts and realize that we aren't in it alone. If you are an ex- spouse reading this book, we hope you will find your space, your place in the post-death-of-an-ex process, and perhaps some help for dealing with your children's grieving and coping processes. We hope you will also consider sharing your story on our website, www.deathofanex.com, so that others can learn from your experience. Most of all, we hope you find a place of peace and healing on your journey of surviving the death of your ex.

Robyn and Robbie

Appendices

The Art of Grieving Gracefully

Suggestions for Coping with Loss and Pain
© Robbie Davis-Floyd

My daughter, Peyton Elizabeth Floyd, died as the result of a car accident on September 12, 2000, four days before her 21st birthday. These are some of the things I learned from the experience of coping with this devastating loss. They begin with suggestions for the immediate period after a loved one's death, and move on to the different coping methods I found useful over the long-term. At the end, I include suggestions for what to say (and not to say) to those who are bereaved.

In the Immediate Aftermath of the News

Drink LOTS of water. If you get dehydrated, you won't be able to cope with anything.

Even if you can hardly swallow, eat a little bit of healthy food at mealtimes. Junk food and soft drinks will only weaken you and compromise your ability to function.

Cry a LOT. Every tear carries stress hormones out of your body. The more you cry, the more capable you will be of standing up to life in the midst of your grief.

Take every opportunity to laugh that comes your way. Laughter stimulates your immune system, which helps to keep you healthy. Every moment of joy and laughter you experience will remind you for a little while that life can still be worth living.

Later, When You Have Time

Read about grief and shock. Learning about the symptoms that others have experienced helps you know you are normal and not going crazy when your grief is so deep and your pain so intense that you can hardly see two feet in front of you, because of the fog of agony that surrounds you.

The physical components of grief can be stunning in the first months or year—like a butcher knife in the heart, daggers in your back, a hole blown in your stomach. Know that level of intensity will pass. You may always feel pain, but it won't be as horrible, and over time, amazingly enough, you can learn to live with it. While it lasts, let your friends cocoon you as often as you can. Sometimes, when you are with people who surround you with love, the butcher knife will come out of your heart for a little while. It will go back in, but less and less deeply over time.

Don't hesitate to name the person you lost and talk about him or her when appropriate in conversation. If it makes others uncomfortable, simply state that you need to talk about your loved one in a normal way, and that you will deeply appreciate their understanding. They will rise to it and find that they are relieved as well. Nothing is more awkward than skirting around the issue that is on everyone's mind—the elephant in the room—best to just put it right out there.

Tell your story as often as you can in appropriate times and places. Narrating a tragic event helps you to get that it happened, to give it form and focus in your mind, and eventually may help you find some meaning in it all. To people who want to "do something for you," explain that the most loving thing they can do is *listen to your story*.

When you are telling your story, or talking about your tragedy, do so appropriately. Don't take more than your fair share of others' time and attention. I call this "the art of grieving gracefully." If you talk or cry for too long, everyone else gets very uncomfortable. You will feel their tension, and you will become uncomfortable too. There is no healing in talking when others don't want to hear it anymore—it will just make you feel worse in the end.

Experience and process grief whenever it bubbles up inside you. Grief is *hard work* that must be done for your own mental health. You can only do the work of grief healthily if you go through it, leaning into the pain. Your grief may accompany you throughout the rest of your life, causing you enormous pain, but also making you far stronger than you could ever imagine.[1] As long as you grieve, you will still be able to experience joy and happiness—they are opposite sides of the same coin, powerful emotions that require you to *feel* in order to experience them. Refusing to grieve will diminish your ability to feel other emotions and to show up to life.

Metaphorically speaking, grief is like a river—*it has to flow*. Sometimes it will rise up like a tidal wave and take you

---

1   A caveat here: Yes, suffering can make you stronger. But prolonged suffering can also make you a great deal weaker. Years of grieving and sorrow can take their toll on our immune systems and psychological resilience, especially when an initial huge loss is compounded by multiple future losses. In the 9 years after my daughter died, my fiancé broke up with me, other loved ones died, my house burned down, and I had an astonishingly painful total knee replacement. The cumulative effect of those multiple stressors (and there were many more) left me drained and depleted, unable to carry on with my life. So I checked myself into rehab at the fabulous Sierra Tuscon residential treatment facility. Diagnosed there with "trauma, anxiety, and depression," I took a full month off from daily life to focus on healing myself and regaining my energy and resilience, and it worked! (For descriptions of some of my experiences there, see *The Power of Ritual* by Robbie Davis-Floyd and Charles Laughlin, Daily Grail Press, 2016.)

down. At those times, just let it—find someplace private and, if possible, someone to support you, and sob all you need to—scream, yell, pound pillows—just surrender to the grief. It can be terrifying to feel that depth of emotion, but the more you let it flow, the faster the tidal wave will pass through you. You will be amazed at how much better you feel after it has passed.

At other times, grief is like a waterfall that suddenly and quickly cascades over you. This grief cascade often happens when you get unexpectedly blindsided by, for example, seeing a person that looks just like your loved one, or coming up out of a subway and finding yourself near the street where they lived, or seeing a book they loved, or hearing an expression they often used. If you know such things are coming, you can psychologically prepare for them and avoid the sudden cascade of pain, but often things just happen and suddenly, you are overwhelmed. Just go with it and cry for a while—it will pass.

Sometimes the river of grief flows still and deep—you know grief is happening inside you but you are granted space to live your life and get on with your work. Such times are gifts—use them well without any guilt that you are not honoring your loved one enough by staying miserable. When the tidal wave or the waterfall takes you down again, flow with it, and know that gradually, you will come back up and have room to breathe again for a while.

If you try to dam up your grief, please know that it will eventually smash your dam and take you down anyway. If you try to prevent that, you may well end up drinking or taking drugs to dull your pain, and spiral down into a clinical depression. That will be much worse than letting it flow as it will.

Depression is not grief—it is the absence of emotion. Grieving, like joy, is stimulating and healthy for your immune system. Depression is terrible for your immune system and your mental stability—in a depression, you lose your ability to feel anything except pain. I call it "the flatlands." The world seems grey, dull, and flat, pain is all you feel, and suicide starts to seem logical as a way out of the pain. If you find yourself spiraling down into a depression, get help immediately. Some people can stop the onset of depression through exercise, meditation, activities that nurture them, etc., but many of us need antidepressants to stabilize our brain chemicals and stop the downward spiral so we can stabilize and regain our ability to feel, and thus to grieve in a healthy way.

Don't expect to "heal" your grief and pain, or "get over it." You might, and you might not. Just learn to live with it as a part of you. Expecting that by the end of some particular period of time, you should be "all better" just makes you feel worse if you are not. As long as you are willing to let the grief flow, to do the hard work of grieving whenever it bubbles up or cascades over you, then you are where you are supposed to be in your grieving process.

When you spend years loving someone who dies, at what point do you think it will stop seeming like you just saw them yesterday? There may be no such point, and you may find yourself often re-shocked to have to remember that they died. *The power and duration of your grief will mirror the power and duration of your love.* So if you love deeply, don't expect to "get over it." Just learn to live with it, and *honor your ability to love that much.*

Make or keep a special place in your house where you can talk in private to the person you lost, and grieve or laugh or remember at times. A room, or an altar. Fill it with special things that belonged to that person, and handle, hug, or kiss them when you are the saddest and loneliest. In your deepest need and longing, take one of those things to bed with you and cradle it in your arms, or wear it if it's clothing. One or several of those precious objects will bring you the tang of your loved one's presence, like a whiff of salt air that evokes the sea. It's no compensation for the loss of their actual physical presence, but it is better than having nothing at all to hold onto.

Don't keep everything that belonged to your loved one—give everything away that is not especially meaningful to you personally. You may find a lot of pleasure and relief in letting family or friends of your loved one choose special things that will help them in their own grief. But don't give away anything until you are ready, and be sure you are willing to let it go before you give it. You don't need any more wrenches, so wait until the gift to another is not a wrench, but a gift to you.

Talk, pray, or write letters to the one you lost—perhaps on your laptop or in a journal. Just because they are physically dead does not mean that their spirit cannot hear you. Assume that they are listening, and say to them whatever is in your heart, even angry things. It can be useful to believe, or imagine, that they hear you and understand, and will help you if they can.

If miracles happen, like your loved one coming to you in a vision or dream, or sending you a message, write them down immediately so you won't forget that they happened. Don't expect miracles, but be present and aware and grateful if they occur.

Find a good balance between spending time with others and spending time alone. Sometimes you need company, and sometimes grief-work is best done by yourself alone. When you receive an invitation or are expected somewhere, listen to yourself and do what will nurture you the most.

Never negate the existence of your dead loved one in order to be polite. For example, if you've lost a child, when new acquaintances ask you if you have children, just speak the truth. I tried a couple of times to say, "Yes, I have a son, Jason," and then I felt as if I had just completely erased my daughter, Peyton's, life. So now I say, in a light tone, "Yes, I raised two kids. My daughter, Peyton, was killed in a car accident some years ago, and my son, Jason, is now 31 and doing great!" Then quickly change the subject by asking the other person some light-hearted question, so that they won't feel obliged to dwell on your child's death unless they really want to, and the conversation can move on. It doesn't help you or them to make a big deal of it at an initial, casual meeting. Same for the death of any other loved one.

Be very gentle with yourself. If you are not getting as much work done as you think you should, celebrate each thing that you do accomplish. Don't watch tragic movies, turn off the news if it hurts you to hear it, read books that are joyful and fun, spend time in the sunlight, and get massages as often as you can. If stories of others' tragedies hurt you, don't listen to them. If people give you dumb advice or suggestions that hurt your feelings (such as, "It's time to get over it and move on with your life"), just politely ignore them and change the subject. Or if you have the strength, educate them about what a grieving person really needs. Here are some suggestions from a group in Austin called "For the Love of Christi":

- Please don't ask me if I am over it yet. I'll never get over it.

- Please don't tell me she's in a better place—she isn't here with me.

- Please don't say at least she isn't suffering—I haven't come to terms with why she had to suffer at all, and I am suffering now.

- Please don't tell me you know how I feel unless you have experienced the same kind of loss.

- Please don't ask if I feel better—bereavement is not a condition that clears up.

- Please don't tell me, "at least you had her all those years." What year would you choose for your loved one to die?

- Please don't tell me God never gives us more than we can bear. I don't believe I can bear this pain.

- Please, just say you are sorry. Just say you remember my loved one, if you do. Mention his name. Listen to my story. Or just let me cry.

From my heart and the depths of my own pain over losing my father, mother, mother-in-law, 20-year-old daughter, sister-in-law, some very close friends, and most recently my ex-husband, I ask you to remember that *"what you resist, persists."* So when you are sure you can't go on for one more day or minute, express your despair to anyone who will listen, insist that you *can't* as many times as you need to, cry, or scream as much as you feel like doing. When you have fully expressed your resistance, despair, and certainty that you can't go on, then deep down inside yourself, where the spirit of your loved one(s) will always dwell, you will find the strength you need.

What To Say To Those Who Lose Loved Ones, and What Not To Say

(I think I must have adapted some of the following from a flyer passed out by For the Love of Christi—or perhaps from some of its meetings that I attended—and some of it is my own. I can no longer remember which is which!)

"You'll be with him again in Heaven." Very not helpful. We want them right here, right now! It does us a great deal more good for you to acknowledge that. If, in fact, we will meet them again, we will come to that faith in our own time. Don't push it, just let us know that you recognize our pain.

"I can imagine what you are going through." No, you can't if you haven't gone through it yourself. So don't go there, it makes us want to hit you!

"I can't imagine what you are going through." Better to hear, because it's true and it makes us not resentful of your presumption, but grateful that you recognize that indeed you can't imagine—neither could we.

Please, let us talk about our dead loved ones, let us tell stories about them, give us every opportunity you can to mention their names. There is enormous relief for me in just saying "Peyton," or "Robert," and even more relief in telling stories about things they said and did the way others do about their living kids or exes without anybody acting weird. The very greatest gift you can give a grieving person, especially in the first two years after the death, is to ask us to tell our stories of loss. *But please, if you do ask, then be prepared to listen.*

Choose your timing well. Don't ask a bereaved person to tell their story when you have no time to hear it. Don't offer condolences when that person is walking to the stage to give a speech, or is about to attend an important meeting! And don't worry about re-opening a wound—this wound never closes—but do it at a time when we can go into it with you and really talk about it, not in passing on the street.

Narrating an event is the most powerful way to give it coherence and meaning. It is devastating to be asked to tell the story of your loved one's death, to start telling the story (which means re-experiencing it as if it were happening right now), and then to be interrupted with questions like "Why didn't you do this or that?" or with calls to the waiter or whatever. We know you have limited time and energy—just give us free rein and let us tell you the story as it comes out, without interruption (pertinent questions always welcome). Know as you listen that we are giving you the greatest gift we can by sharing the greatest pain we hold, and you are giving us the greatest gift you have by listening to our stories and acknowledging our pain. You don't have to try to fix anything, *just listen* and give us the gift of *being heard*! If you are not prepared to go there, don't even broach the subject beyond the bare minimum of "I'm sorry for your loss."

The other side of that coin is that sometimes the bereaved one is feeling okay in that moment, and may not really want to talk about it at all. Let them know you are open to hearing their story, but if they are not up for talking about it, respect their need not to go there at that time. As time moves on, I find myself less and less willing to plunge into my pain in front of others, while for the first 3 years after my daughter died, and the first few months after my ex died, I was desperate for opportunities to do that.

Yet, sometimes I still want that kind of attention, and now that it has been over 14 years since Peyton died, and 3 years after the death of my ex, almost nobody wants to talk with me about any of that any more. When I bring up my daughter or my ex in casual conversation, perhaps sharing childhood or marriage stories with friends, they don't follow up my stories with further questions, as you would if the child or the ex were still alive. That's hard. I want to talk about them in a normal way, want people to ask me what Peyton was like, how she grew up, what she was into, and what Robert was like, how was our marriage, how is it for me to lose an ex I loved.

So please, when you talk to a bereaved person, don't stiffen when the subject of their loved one comes up—just relax and go with the flow. And sometimes, just sometimes, ask us how we really are, how hard has it really been, would we share with you how we have managed to get through? If it's the right time, your questions will be manna to our souls, and our answers can help us to feel proud that we have made it this far.

Appendix 2

RESOURCES FOR SURVIVING THE DEATH OF YOUR EX

Three places you should consider calling or visiting if you have children who were affected:

1. **The funeral home** that arranged your ex-spouse's funeral can be a great resource for finding local therapists or grief resources. Many funeral homes that employ therapists will also offer grief counseling that is free or at a reduced rate for immediate family. Some even offer programs or a contact person to help your children through the funeral and burial process.

2. **Your child's school counselors** are an excellent resource to put you in touch with community-based programs. It can also be helpful to have someone at school that can "watch over" your child and work with them as they move through the grief process.

3. **The Social Security Administration:** Your children (and potentially you—even as an ex) may be eligible for survivor benefits. Please take the time to read these publications and visit your local Social Security Administration offices: http://www.ssa.gov

SSA Publication No. 05-10008, ICN 451390, November 2009, and *How Social Security Can Help You When A Family Member Dies* http://www.ssa.gov/pubs/10008.html

Also recommended

1. **The State Bar** if you need help finding a good probate attorney (especially if your ex did not have a will). Probate can be a difficult course to navigate and it is helpful to have someone who can look after the best interests of your children in respect to your ex's estate.

2. Visit our website, www.deathofanex.com, for more resources and stories as they are made available to us.

Take Care of Yourself

• Read Robbie's Appendix on coping with grief, and seek out additional resources.

• Buy a notebook and keep a private journal—it's amazing how much healing you can find on a piece of paper.

• Find a point person you can call or reach out to. Make sure that he or she is also someone who will intervene if you are going down the rabbit hole.

Find a Support Group

GriefShare Resources, Support Group Directory
http://www.griefshare.org/

The Dougy Center—The National Center for Grieving Children & Families Resources, Support Group Directory Primarily for Children
http://www.dougy.org/grief-support-programs/

Foundation for Grieving Children Resources, Support Group Directory for Children
http://www.foundationforgrievingchildren.org/blog

For the Love of Christi, a grief center in Austin, Texas dealing with all kinds of grief
> http://fortheloveofchristi.org/

Grief Recovery Online (founded by) Widows and Widowers Online Support Group for All
> http://www.groww.org/

Alliance of Hope for Suicide Survivors Resources, Online Support Group for Suicide Survivors
> http://www.allianceofhope.org/

American Association of Suicidology Resources, Support Group Directory for Suicide Survivors
> http://www.suicidology.org/suicide-support-group-directory

Grief Resource Directories

Grief Speaks Comprehensive listing of grief resources and groups
> www.griefspeaks.com

Grief Support Resources for Children Rainbows
> http://www.rainbows.org/

National Alliance for Grieving Children
> http://childrengrieve.org/

Grief Support Resources for Military Families Tragedy Assistance Program for Survivors
> http://www.taps.org

Biographies

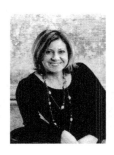

ROBYN HASS is a very happily re-married wife and mom to two young boys and three beautiful step-daughters. After completing a double master's degree in social work and public health in 2002, Robyn began working for an international firm providing public health and business management consulting to various high-profile clients, including the U.S. Department of Defense. She has since "retired" from the consulting world, and she and her husband now own a small business together.

In *Surviving the Death of Your Ex*, Robyn shares the very personal account of the tragic and unexpected death of her recently divorced ex-husband, and the mountains of grief she had to climb with her young son as they worked through his loss. As a trained and degreed therapist, Robyn was familiar with loss and grief, but nothing prepared her for the plethora of mixed emotions that surfaced after his death—emotions that no one talked about. As she searched for professional literature on the subject, she realized very little existed and what was published was almost completely unavailable to the general public. She felt this had to change, and along with her co-editor Robbie Davis-Floyd, she set out to bring the subject to a larger audience and find ways to help grieving ex-spouses heal. Along the way, they found many others in similar situations and invited them to share their stories.

Robyn, her husband Joseph, and their two boys currently reside in the piney woods of east Texas, just outside of Houston. She can be contacted at info@deathofanex.com.

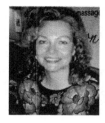 ROBBIE DAVIS-FLOYD, PHD, Senior Research Fellow, Dept. of Anthropology, University of Texas Austin, and Fellow of the Society for Applied Anthropology, is a devoted mother to her son, Jason, an adoring friend to her daughter-in-law, Ashley, and is over the moon about being a grandmother to Jaxon Wallace Floyd, age 4, Robert Grayson Floyd, age 2, and Shayla Ann Hall, age 8. After completing a PhD in Anthropology and Folklore at the University of Texas Austin in 1986, she embarked on a long teaching and public-speaking career, focusing on the anthropology of reproduction, childbirth, midwifery, and obstetrics, as well as on ritual and symbolic studies. She is an internationally renowned speaker in those arenas, author of over 80 published articles, and author, co-author, or lead editor for 10 volumes, including *Birth as an American Rite of Passage*; *Childbirth and Authoritative Knowledge: Cross-Cultural Perspectives*; *From Doctor to Healer: The Transformative Journey*, *Birth Models That Work*; and most recently, *The Power of Ritual*.

This book constitutes for Robbie a departure from her usual endeavors. She welcomed the opportunity to collaborate with Robyn when they mutually discovered that they both wanted to write about their experiences of dealing with the deaths of their ex-husbands, and to find others who wished to do the same. They share a strong passion for hearing women's voices and providing a forum for their stories. That shared passion has resulted in this book.

Robbie and her family currently reside in Austin, Texas, widely regarded by its residents as "the music capital of the world" and "the center of the known universe." We heartily agree! Robbie can be contacted at davis-floyd@austin.utexas.edu.

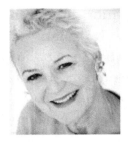

Now retired, KIRSTEN DEHNER has spent the last eight years enjoying single life in the vibrant ex-pat community of San Miguel de Allende, a historically rich pueblo in the high desert plateau nestled in the Sierra Madres of central Mexico. She maintains close touch with her two children living in the States, Marah Abel and Josh Abel. Kirsten has a B.A. in painting from UCLA, and is an MFA graduate of the Creative Writing/ Fiction program at Columbia University, where she was editor of the university's literary journal. She also had a brief career as a professional actor. At Synapse Technologies, Inc., L.A., her ex-husband Bob Abel's company, she served as senior writer, associate creative director, and segment producer on two multi-million-dollar (pre-Internet) interactive multimedia IBM educational projects: *Columbus: Encounter, Discovery and Beyond* (now in the Library of Congress); and *Evolution/Revolution: The World Discovers Itself (1890-1930)*. At Synapse, she was also involved in digital domain designs, and BUB: Books UnBound, an interactive book prototype.

In 1995, Kirsten created one of the Internet's first (and still operating) bilingual sites, a consumer health information site, NOAH: New York Online Access to Health, for CUNY's Research Foundation, The New York Public Library, and The New York Academy of Medicine. Under various capacities and titles, and as a freelancer, she has worked in Citibank's marketing department, SoftWatch, Inc., Barnard College, Tom Nicholson & Associates. In San Miguel, Kirsten returned to acting with a one-woman show, several lead roles, and two director credits. She has had an ambivalent relationship with her own writing, but writing about her first ex-husband's death proved so meaningful that she can say it has put her back into a groove long neglected.

ANNETTE BIRCHARD (pseud) is, first and foremost, a mother to a beautiful 22-year-old daughter. She received a Computer Science degree from the University of Iowa in 1981, and has spent the last 30 years as a software developer for many business-diverse companies. Recently, her career goals have changed—they now include making a difference in people's lives. She is actively pursuing a Masters Degree in Gerontology from the University of Nebraska. With her contribution to *Surviving the Death of Your Ex*, Annette shares her personal account of the brutal murder of her ex-husband, and the tremendous amount of anger she experienced around *what could have been* regarding her relationship with her ex-husband. She also shares her anger toward her step-daughters, and the grief of her daughter—who considered her step-father to be one of the most influential people in her life.

"After the murder of my ex-husband, I searched online for information on how to help myself and my daughter, but I didn't find very much material. This book will provide a valuable resource for those who have experienced the death of an ex-spouse. In the 21ˢᵗ century, blended families are common, and resources to help surviving ex-spouses and children are desperately needed."

~

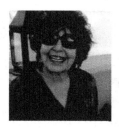

CAROL EINHORN WHEELER was, for many years, a magazine editor and writer in New York City. She began at *Savvy* magazine when it first started in 1978 (which was when she and her first husband split up). At *Savvy*, Carol did many interviews, a plethora of book reviews, regular fashion and beauty pieces, and anything else that needed doing. The next magazine she worked at was *Woman's Day*, where she was a features editor and a copywriter. At *Executive Female*, a women's business magazine, she was executive editor, and wrote and edited full-length features, as well as short pieces. Sometime later, when she moved to Sag Harbor for a while, she tried another kind of journalism, at a weekly— the *East Hampton Star*.

After the death of her beloved second husband, she decided to leave New York, the enchanted city, and move to a different country. She is now a resident of San Miguel de Allende, Mexico. She welcomed (with some misgivings) the opportunity to write about the horrible ending of her first marriage. It was a subject she'd always wanted to cover, but unfortunately, it required reliving the worst experiences in her life, so until Robbie and Robyn offered a framework, she was unable to do it. It was also helpful to realize that many women had had similar experiences, in that they found themselves looking at their divorced husbands in a different light later in life, and particularly after the ex had died. The subject seems to evoke a companionable feeling and a recognition among many women, in fact. But until this book was proposed, I don't think many of us realized how universal a feeling it is. Nevertheless, Carol still can't read over the chapter she wrote without weeping. Asked about what keeps her busy these days, Carol replied, "I cry a lot."

~

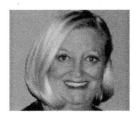

MELANIE has been very happily married to the love of her life for 30 years. Although she encountered some serious "bumps" in her late teens with an unexpected pregnancy, she found a way to put herself through nursing school, starting at the age of 17. She has been a successful nurse for 34 years. Her married life to a U.S. Air Force officer took her and her two sons around the world, and enabled her to garner knowledge in various areas of nursing. Yet, she discovered when her "baby daddy" died that none of her nursing knowledge of the grief process or life experiences had prepared her to handle that event, which turned out to be one of the hardest situations that she and her son had ever experienced. Melanie wanted to share her experience of dealing with the feelings her son went through at the time of his estranged birth parent's sudden death. She is now aware this situation is not uncommon. There are now many "baby daddies" who have no relationship with the children they helped to create, yet suddenly enter their abandoned children's lives when they die. No one is ever really prepared for death, much less facing the death of someone from a difficult past, who left Melanie and her son when he was a newborn. His death thrust them both harshly into the world of the "sins of the father." Melanie quickly found out that there weren't any resources available to help her through. As an unwed teenage mother, her parents had completely turned their back on her at her son's birth, and therefore, she had no family support to fall back on during a very difficult time when family support was greatly needed. She wants other women to know that they can be stronger than they ever thought possible.

Melanie is now a retired nurse and enjoys sharing time with the many friends she has the privilege of having made this far in her journey through life. She takes pride that she will be a "hippie at heart" for the rest of the time she has left on Planet Earth. Melanie and her husband, Michael, currently reside in South Texas, living near to her two now-married sons. She has three beautiful grandchildren. She can be reached at mimejeexp@gmail.com.

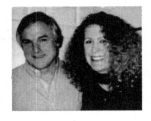

LAURIE WIMMER, a 23-year veteran of Oregon politics, is a Government Relations Consultant for the Oregon Education Association. In her 17 years with OEA, Laurie has become a policy specialist on school finance and taxation, education alternatives, health and safety issues, and community college funding. Laurie has served as an appointee to various policy work groups.

She is the co-founder and chair of the Oregon Revenue Coalition. She has also served as Vice Chair of the School District Business Best Practices Advisory Committee (on school district performance audits), as a member of the School Revenue Forecast Committee, and on various educational choice groups, including the Charter School Task Force, the Virtual School Advisory Committee of the Department of Education, and the 10-year-review committee on Oregon's charter school law. She has written and produced for OEA an Annotated Glossary of School Finance and Taxation and co-authored for the Revenue Coalition a Primer on Tax Expenditures.

Prior to her work with OEA, she served for six years as Executive Director of the Oregon Commission for Women, where she helped to pass historic legislation on family leave, stalking, sexual harassment, domestic relations law, and women's health policy. Laurie has been a writer and editor for 30 years. Her work has been published in international, national, and local publications, including *Black Lamb, Zephyr Magazine,* and *Willamette Week.* Laurie is an honors graduate of Vassar College. She interned with the Project on Equal

Education Rights, and the New York Public Interest Research Group, while at Vassar. Laurie lives in northwest Portland with her two foster children, Akili, 12, and Amina, 17. She also has two biological children—Griffin, 23, and Riley, 20 who are completing their college studies. She is currently the President of her class at Vassar, and Secretary of the Board of Oregon's Virtual Education program through the NW Regional ESD. She has also served as an advisor to the Constitution Team at Parkrose High School, as President of the Vassar Club of Oregon, and as Chair of the board of directors of Emerge Oregon. She sleeps on alternate Sundays.

~

ALYESHKA HARMON (pseud) counts her children and her friends as two of the greatest blessings in her life.

She finds women's stories endlessly fascinating, and she is honored to be included in this volume. Alyeshka believes that what happens to us becomes our story, and then we become stewards of our stories. It is up to us to know when to share them, and with whom, because our stories are medicine, and they can teach or encourage others. She first discovered the healing power of stories in her early thirties, when she was told she had two years left to live. She searched for stories of people who had overcome "terminal" diagnoses, knowing that if she could find just one such story, it would be enough. She found several, and then went on to make her own healing story.

Alyeshka has degrees from Harvard, University of Chicago, and Johns Hopkins. She is at work on the early stages of a collection of true stories from women who have survived extraordinary situations.

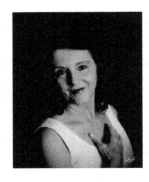

Rima Star has a BA from Texas Lutheran University and a Master's degree in Sociology and Political Science from the University of Houston; she also studied secondary teaching and educational counseling at Texas State University. She has thousands of hours of experience, education, and training in body-mind-spirit integrative and holistic modalities, including massage therapy, breath therapy, and doula work. She trained in midwifery and labor support (1984-85) with Marimikel Potter, RN, CPM, in Austin. She visited the former Soviet Union (1988) to speak, teach, and meet with families and birth professionals who pioneered water birth in that country. She founded the Star Institute (1998-2006) to provide curricula in education for birth, health, and creative living. She has worked in education, government, and business. Rima developed and taught Ebb and Flow Integration Therapy™ and the Birth Journey Facilitator Program™. Now she is the founder and CEO of O3 Skincare™ topical ozone products. Rima is author of *The Healing Power of Birth*. A portion of proceeds from product sales goes to support the "Saving Water Birth History" project, and the publication of her book, *Water Birth Wisdom*. She has attended and spoken at numerous birth, midwifery, and pre- and perinatal psychology conventions. Rima was given an award (2004) as a "Mother of Water Birth" in the United States, and in 2009 as a "Pioneer of Massage Therapy." She says:

> *My work is dedicated to bringing hope, help, and healing hands to families, individuals, and professionals–anyone who has been born. I see*

each day as "a new birth"—for each of us—and an opportunity to make the choices, and our strongest movement, toward whatever makes our hearts sing. Currently, I am settling into the experience of having a married daughter, gaining a son-in-law, and becoming a grandmother. To write on the passing of one of the loves of my life, and the healing of years of non-communication with him, to once again be present with him in his last three years, is a rewarding experience. I believe we must constantly re-view our stories and ask if there's another way we see that story now. I'm grateful for the opportunity to do that and share my experience with you.

She can be reached through her website www.RimaStar.com or at info@RimaStar.com.

Made in the USA
Columbia, SC
07 April 2020

90650286R00153